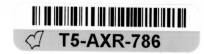

REFUSAL TO SPEAK

REFUSAL TO SPEAK

TREATMENT OF SELECTIVE MUTISM IN CHILDREN

Sheila A. Spasaro, Ph.D.
and
Charles E. Schaefer, Ph.D.
editors

A JASON ARONSON BOOK

ROWMAN & LITTLEFIELD PUBLISHERS, INC.
Lanham • Boulder • New York • Toronto • Oxford

A JASON ARONSON BOOK

ROWMAN & LITTLEFIELD PUBLISHERS, INC.

Published in the United States of America
by Rowman & Littlefield Publishers, Inc.
A wholly owned subsidiary of The Rowman & Littlefield Publishing Group, Inc.
4501 Forbes Boulevard, Suite 200, Lanham, Maryland 20706
www.rowmanlittlefield.com

PO Box 317
Oxford
OX2 9RU, UK

British Library Cataloguing in Publication Information Available

Library of Congress Cataloging-in-Publication Data

Refusal to speak: treatment of selective mutism in children/Sheila Spasaro and Charles
Schaefer, editors.
    p. cm.
  Includes bibliographical references and index.
  ISBN 0-7657-0125-1 (alk. paper)
  1. Mutism, Elective—Treatment. I. Spasaro, Sheila. II. Schaefer, Charles E.
RJ506.M87R44 1998
618.92'89—dc21   97-40384

Printed in the United States of America

CONTENTS

PART II: BEHAVIOR THERAPY

PART III: PSYCHODYNAMIC THERAPY

PART IV: PSYCHOPHARMACOLOGIC APPROACHES

PART V: GROUP AND FAMILY THERAPY

PART VI: MULTIMODAL TREATMENT

PREFACE

SELECTIVE MUTISM IN children is characterized by a persistent refusal to speak in one or more social situations, despite the ability to use and comprehend language. Children manifesting this disorder speak normally at home but refuse to speak in school or to strangers. Although the symptoms of the disorder may be apparent in preschool years, a child with selective mutism does not generally come to clinical attention until he or she enters school.

In the past, selective mutism has been known for its resistance to treatment. More recently, however, the range of treatment options has expanded to include promising behavioral, psychopharmacological, and multimodal approaches. This volume, comprehensive in scope, presents the major therapeutic approaches that have been reported in the literature to date. The basic premise of the book is that clinicians who are both familiar with the various treatment options and skilled in their application will best be able to individualize their strategies to meet the needs of an individual case.

In recent years, there has been a growing trend for therapists to combine and integrate techniques and theoretical concepts in clinical practice. The goal of such an eclectic, multicomponent approach as applied to selective mutism is to strengthen treatment efficacy and overcome the traditional intractability of the disorder. An additional trend is for clinicians to follow a prescriptive approach wherein the selection of a treatment for a particular disorder, such as selective mutism, is guided by the extant literature. This volume provides practical information regarding treatment options and outcomes to the practicing clinician who is actively treating children.

Refusal to Speak: Treatment of Selective Mutism in Children is divided into six sections. The chapters contained within the sections discuss assessment and treatment planning options as well as behavioral, psychodynamic, psychopharmacological, group and family, and multicomponent approaches to treatment. This book should be of interest to clinicians and students from diverse disciplines, including psychology, psychiatry, pediatrics, counseling, and social work.

1

AN INTRODUCTION TO THE TREATMENT OF SELECTIVE MUTISM

*Sheila A. Spasaro, Jessica Platt,
and Charles E. Schaefer*

DESCRIPTION OF THE DISORDER

For decades, clinicians have encountered selectively mute children in their practices. Often these children are brought into treatment by parents who report that their child refuses to speak in all but the most familiar situations, despite the child's adequate verbal skills. Teacher reports of these children frequently indicate that they are average or above average in intelligence. Indeed, selectively mute children may succeed in school despite their resistance to verbal behavior. Parents report that the child's language developed normally, but he or she became increasingly shy with strangers. Often, the parents are not aware that there is a problem until the child enters school and the refusal to speak is reported by the teacher. It is at this point that the selectively mute child may come to the attention of a pediatrician or mental health professional.

Parents may be baffled by reports of their child's refusal to speak since selectively mute children continue to communicate at home to family members and other familiar individuals. This discrepancy between the child's private and public behavior is so troubling to parents that they sometimes bring tapes of the child's speech within the family to teachers and clinicians to prove that he or she does, indeed, speak at home.

Examples of this interesting clinical phenomenon have existed in the literature since 1877, when Kussmaul first described cases of *aphasia voluntaria*, but it is Tramer (1934) who is credited with first using the term *elective mutism* to describe this clinical presentation. The name of the disorder was changed to *selective mutism* (SM) with publication of the *Diagnostic and Statistical Manual of Mental Disorders* (*DSM-IV*; American Psychiatric Association [APA] 1994). Selective mutism is characterized by a persistent failure to speak in nonfamiliar social situations where there is an expectation of speech, for example, at school, although the individual has demonstrated an ability to speak in other situations. This refusal to speak in nonfamiliar situations interferes with the functioning of the child and lasts for a period of at least one month, not limited to the first month of school. Selective mutism generally has its onset before the age of 5, although the child is typically not referred to a clinician until the time of entry into school, perhaps because the level of impairment is not clear until this transition into the nonfamiliar school environment. Selective mutism is a relatively rare disorder, accounting for fewer than 1 percent of persons seen in mental health settings (APA 1994). Evidence of the rarity of the disorder is provided by earlier studies reporting prevalence rates for selective mutism (e.g., Bradley and Sloman 1975, Fundudis et al. 1979).

The integrity of this diagnostic category is not without challenge. The discussion typically centers around the category's overlap in expression with features of several anxiety-spectrum disorders, specifically, social phobia, simple phobia, and obsessive-compulsive disorder (e.g., Black and Uhde 1992, Boon 1994, Crumley 1990, 1993), as well as with disorders characterized by negative, manipulative, controlling, and oppositional behavior (Browne et al. 1963, Kolvin and Fundudis 1981, Rosenberg and Lindblad 1978, Wright and Cuccaro 1994).

Other authors have described the selective mute's anxiety as related phenomenologically to the borderline or psychotic-spectrum disorders (Atlas 1993). Atlas emphasized the selective mute's tenuous experience of the self as different from but existing within the surrounding environment. Therapeutic work is therefore directed toward enhancing the child's overall psychological integrity. Jacobsen (1995) proposed that, in cases of severe abuse or trauma, selective mutism may be associated with a diagnosis of dissociative identity disorder (DID) and may be a part of its polysymptomatic presentation. In this case report, the patient did not make significant progress until DID was diagnosed and treated. Jacobsen pointed out, however, that this case was atypical in that the onset of mutism occurred in adolescence rather than prior to age 5, and its duration was years, rather than months, long. In addition, speech was censored by selected identity states. It appears that the mutism described here may be qualitatively different from the preponderance of cases of selective mutism.

There is also discussion in the literature of the difference between selective mutism and what has been called progressive or total mutism. A distinction is drawn between children who select to whom, when, and where they will speak, that is, selective mutism, and those who do not speak to anyone at all, that is, total mutism (Marcus et al. 1993, Paniagua and Saeed 1987, 1988). Marcus and colleagues described the use of multiple clinical techniques to elicit significant improvement in an 11-year-old boy who was totally mute. Interventions included contingency management, modeling, social skills training, and the use of white noise to diminish anxiety in the presence of speech phobia. Despite these very varied clinical presentations, the diagnostic integrity of SM has been maintained and refined in *DSM-IV* (APA 1994) from its former category of elective mutism (*DSM-III-R*; [APA 1987]).

ETIOLOGY

Several rationales have been proposed as etiologically significant in the development of selective mutism. Psychodynamic explanations have associated the symptomatology of selective mutism with psy-chosexual-phase conflicts and regression to or fixation at an earlier developmental stage (Browne et al. 1963, Radford 1977). Other psychodynamic authors emphasized the complex meaning of the silence itself, as a symptom that synthesizes the conflicts of various developmental levels (Chethik 1973). Silence, according to Chethik, has multiple meanings and functions, not only as a defense, but as a source of intense gratification.

By far, the most common etiological factor noted in the literature, however, is the presence of family psychopathology. There has been a general consensus among authors regarding the basic characteristics of families of selectively mute children (Carr and Afnan 1989). The most prominent of these is the involvement of the mother and child in a symbiotic relationship and the failure of the mother-child dyad to achieve separation and individuation (Clemente et al. 1986). The mother is described as lonely, depressed, and distant, even hostile, in her relationship with the father. The child may not share the mother's hostility toward the father, setting up an ambivalent relationship. The child's relationship with the mother is at once close, dependent, and controlling (Wright 1968). From a family systems perspective, the selective mute's silence may be interpreted as an indirect expression of the mother's hostility and a way to maintain an exclusive relationship with her (Atoynatan 1986). The mother responds to the child's every demand, often even speaking for her. The exclusivity of the relationship, in turn, enables both mother and child to avoid engaging with others. Additional reported characteristics of the mother include passivity and difficulty communicating wants and needs. Indeed, the culture of the home is one in which the open and frank expression of one's feelings is discouraged (Rosenberg and Lindblad 1978). Furthermore, families of selectively mute children are described as socially isolated and possessing rigid, closed boundaries (Lindblad-Goldberg 1986). They are reported to be suspicious and fearful of the world at large. Children from such families are bound by an injunction not to reveal the family's secrets (Baptiste 1995). It should not be surprising, then, that the symptoms of selective mutism often become most pronounced as the family is faced with the task of negotiating a change or transition that involves launching the child into the outside world, such as when the child is entering school.

The exclusive relationship between mother and child seen in selective mutism may result in a fearful, even phobic, response to strangers. Lesser-Katz (1986, 1988) argued that the selective mute's speech inhibition and suppression of motor activity and initiative are similar to the response that other individuals might have to extremely dangerous situations, or to the freeze defense seen in animals. She concluded that this anxious response to strangers belongs, more properly, to an earlier phase of development, and so selective mutism represents a fixation or regression to the stage of infancy. According to Lesser-Katz, one group of these children presents as compliant, timid, passive, and withdrawn, resorting to the freeze defense when in the presence of strangers. Another group of selectively mute children resorts not to the freeze defense but to the fighting reflex when faced with strangers. These children present as noncompliant, passive-aggressive, negativistic, and manipulative. The treatment of choice for both groups involved long-term, nonintrusive therapy aimed at providing the children with a sense of control.

Learning theory suggests an alternative explanation for the development of the disorder, that selective mutism is a learned pattern of behavior that is maintained by reinforcers in the environment. It is, therefore, the principles of classical and operant conditioning, in the form of both positive and negative reinforcement, along with the effects of modeling, that may be responsible for the development of selectively mute behavior (e.g., Marcus et al. 1993). Most of the behavioral literature does not focus on the basis for selective mutism, but rather on the manipulation of current environmental factors in order to increase the child's verbal behavior. Selective mutism is simply a learned pattern of behavior dependent on overt variables. Changing the relationship between the child's speech and the controlling environmental factors can result in more adaptive verbal behavior (Sanok and Ascione 1979). Although studies employing behavioral interventions in the successful treatment of selective mutism provide some empirical evidence for a conceptualization of the disorder based on learning theory (e.g., Nash et al. 1979), it is only one of several possible pathogenic routes. Given the multidimensional conceptualizations of selective mutism in much of the literature, it is difficult to identify a clear etiological course to the disorder.

SELECTED TREATMENT APPROACHES

Several treatment approaches have emerged in the literature, perhaps due to clinicians' divergent thinking about the underlying assumptions regarding the etiology and maintenance of SM. Clinicians attempting to treat this rare and difficult disorder have approached the problem in different ways, and interventions tend to follow psychodynamic, behavioral, or family systems approaches.

PSYCHODYNAMIC TREATMENT

An interesting and technically pure presentation of a psychodynamic intervention was described by Radford (1977) in her treatment of a 6-year-old selectively mute boy named Robert. Conceptualization of the case followed Anna Freud's developmental profile in which attention was directed away from the child's symptomatology and toward his position on a developmental scale with regard to drive, ego, superego, personality structure, primary versus secondary thought processes, and age adequacy of developmental level. Individual psychotherapy was conducted on a once weekly basis for a period of three and a half years. Interpretation of the transference was the main tool of this insight-oriented psychotherapy, which focused on Robert's intrapsychic conflicts. At the time of publication, Robert was speaking in many situations but remained selectively mute in others, although the author pointed out that the mutism was then under conscious control. The aim of the psychotherapy was met, according to Radford, in that it brought about dynamic change in the personality and not merely a reduction in symptomatology.

Chethik (1973) reported on his two-year treatment of Amy, a 6½-year-old selectively mute child. Amy remained silent in the therapy throughout the treatment period, although she began speaking in school and with friends. Communication within the therapy was through drawing, writing, play, body gestures, and sounds. Despite her apparent improvement, that is, a reduction in speech inhibition in other areas of Amy's life at the termination of treatment, Chethik remained concerned that her ego functioning was not free from conflict and regression, which might surface under the stress of adolescence, thus reversing the ego achievements gained in therapy. Clearly, this is a shortcoming of the therapeutic process as is the duration of the treatment itself, which places an enormous burden on the family's resources, straining its emotions, finances, and limited time.

BEHAVIORAL TREATMENT

The preponderance of empirical support in the literature has been for behavioral treatment approaches to selective mutism. Various contingency management procedures have been shown to be successful in increasing verbal behavior in selectively mute children. Successful behavioral interventions with selectively mute children include contingency management, utilizing both positive reinforcers and aversive techniques, transfer of stimulus control and stimulus fading, shaping, self-modeling, and desensitization (Croghan and Craven 1982, Lipton 1980, Matson et al. 1992, Piersel and Kratochwill 1981, Rasbury 1974, Richards and Hansen 1978, Sanok and Streifel 1979, Scott 1977, Van Der Kooy and Webster 1975, Watson and Kramer 1992, Williamson et al. 1977).

Rasbury combined the principles of classical and operant conditioning in her successful treatment of an 11-year-old girl who had been selectively mute since the occurrence of an aversive incident on a school bus six years earlier. The treatment involved construction of a fear hierarchy and in vivo desensitization to speech while the child was transported to school each day by the father. Verbal behavior was positively reinforced by allowing the child to participate in classroom activities of her choosing during the day. There were 140 daily sessions of 10-minute duration and fifteen steps in the hierarchy. Speech was reinstated in the school setting and generalized to other areas of the child's life. The procedure was notable for its use of nonprofessionals (i.e., the father and classroom teacher) for delivery of the actual treatment. Furthermore, the author reported, "Many of the most helpful suggestions throughout the course of treatment were provided by the child's father and teacher. Thus, our involvement was clearly a two-way street in which professional and non-professional contributed equally to the development of a successful therapeutic procedure" (p. 104).

A study of twenty-five selectively mute children sought to examine the differential effectiveness of individual behavioral therapy and a standard school-based remedial program (Sluckin et al. 1991). Behavioral treatment techniques included situation and person fading and use of play to shape the child's speech by rewarding successive approximations. The remedial program consisted of contact with a clinic where the child was seen by special-needs teachers. Results indicated that those children receiving behavioral treatment were more likely to have improved at follow-up.

Another behavioral intervention, implemented in a school setting, was successful in inducing speech in a selectively mute child (Brown and Doll 1988). A whole-class reinforcement system was implemented in which both the child and the other students in her class were allowed to choose prizes any time she spoke to another child in the class. This was later modified so that only the child and the one to whom she spoke were rewarded with a prize. Teacher prompts were used along with a light, which was illuminated whenever the child's speech reached a sufficient loudness. By the end of treatment, the child was speaking in the classroom.

Albert-Stewart (1986) used a tape recorder to provide feedback for positive reinforcement of a selectively mute child who was asked to read into a microphone with speech loud enough to keep a red light illuminated. If the child performed successfully, he was given verbal praise and earned one point. Points were used to purchase a toy. Inaudible speech was ignored. Louder speech was shaped by moving the tape recorder farther and farther away from the child. Spontaneous speech or speech emitted after redirection from the therapist earned five points. The authors noted some loss of progress when the child was simultaneously engaged in psychoanalytically oriented group therapy where the mutism was accepted. When he was subsequently encouraged to speak in the group, there was a recovery of the verbal behavior to the level he had achieved with the behavioral treatment. The authors contended that this case provides evidence of selective mutism as a learned pattern of behavior that is negatively reinforced when there are no expectations for speech.

Self-modeling has been found to be an effective technique for the treatment of selective mutism. For example, Kehle and colleagues (1990) reported a case in which five 5-minute sessions were used to achieve complete remission of symptoms in a selectively mute child. The child was videotaped in the classroom responding to questions asked by his mother. The tape was then edited so that it appeared the child's responses were to the teacher's questioning. The child watched the tape and was rewarded with candy each time it appeared that he had answered one of the teacher's questions. The tape was played to the whole class on the following day, allowing them to learn that the child could, indeed, speak. The procedure was continued with more speech emitted on the tape. Soon the child began conversing with teachers, staff, and peers.

The effectiveness of various behavioral techniques in the treatment of selective mutism has led some researchers to attempt the use of multiple behavioral interventions in treatment of a single case. For example, Watson and Kramer (1992) utilized shaping, multiple reinforcers, natural consequences, stimulus fading, and mild aversives in their treatment of a 9-year-old selectively mute boy. In addition, treatment was delivered both at school and at home. The home intervention produced an increase in verbalization, which generalized to other settings. The school intervention increased the number of people to whom the child spoke, but these results were not maintained at follow-up and did not generalize beyond the training sessions. The authors suggested that possible reasons for this limited success within the school setting included the school's withdrawal from the program before treatment was completed and the staff's acceptance of nonverbal behavior as a means of communication.

On the whole, there is a significant amount of research on the use of behavioral interventions that documents their effectiveness in the treatment of selective mutism. A strength of these interventions is their relative brevity when compared with psychodynamic treatment of selective mutism. Additionally, these studies are both detailed and explicit in their description of the clinical methods used. In most cases, however, the multiple techniques used in many of these reports limit their usefulness since it is not clear which specific interventions are the mechanisms of change.

FAMILY SYSTEMS TREATMENT

Atoynatan (1986) reported on the treatment of seven selectively mute children following a family perspective. In six of the cases, both mother and child received individual psychotherapy. In one case, only the mother was treated. Treatment of the mother was considered an essential component of the therapy since, within this perspective, the dependent mother–child relationship must be resolved if the child is to give up her symptoms. All of the children in this study spoke after a period of one year, with the exception of one who spoke after two years.

Another case study with a selectively mute child documented the use of a family-based intervention focusing on the mother–child relationship (Clemente et al. 1986). An underlying assumption of these authors was that a selectively mute child cannot individuate adequately because her symptoms maintain an unusually close attachment to those from whom she must separate. The mother was seen in individual treatment to work through her hostility toward her immediate family and to come to an understanding of the dysfunctional family dynamics contributing to her daughter's symptoms. The daughter was seen in individual psychodynamically oriented play therapy to establish a positive relationship with another adult, to begin the process of individuation, and to learn to identify and express her ambivalence over resentful and loving feelings toward her mother. The play sessions were unstructured in that the child freely engaged in drawing, playing with dolls, and using a blackboard. The child's brother was also included in many of the sessions to neutralize some of the child's anxiety. Throughout treatment, the mother became less rigid when interacting with her daughter, less anxious about allowing her to form close relationships with others, and more accepting of the child's negative and hostile feelings. The child began to speak freely in school and other settings and improved both academically and socially, as reported by teachers.

Carr and Afnan (1989) reported a case history of a selectively mute child whose treatment implemented a stimulus fading plus reinforcement program. The child was also seen in individual play therapy to reward successive approximations of verbalized play. The stimulus fading consisted of sessions in the school setting with the child's mother and teacher. The child was to read aloud from a book while the distance between mother and child was increased. Reinforcers were dispensed by the father to enhance the connection between them. Within eighteen sessions, the child was regularly speaking to a variety of people.

The family systems approach to the treatment of selective mutism appears to demonstrate some positive results. The approach does, however, make many assumptions about the family's functioning and its contributions to the child's pathology that are unproven. Moreover, since these studies combine many therapeutic techniques, it is not clear that the curative effects are due to delivery of the treatment within a family context.

CONCLUSION

It is difficult to identify a single, most efficacious treatment approach for selective mutism. This book brings together representative examples of successful clinical treatments for the disorder. The studies contained here present effective and practical methods for assessment and treatment of children with SM. While most of the treatments utilize interventions based on theoretical orientations (e.g., behavioral, psychodynamic, systems), several multimodal treatment packages are also presented. As is true in much of the literature on selective mutism, many of the treatments presented here are based on individual case studies or studies of a small number of subjects, which make the results difficult to generalize. The challenge for the future is to design empirical studies that will provide clinicians with reliable evidence about the relative efficacy of our treatments. This is a difficult challenge given the rarity of the disorder, but one we must meet if we are to more fully understand this fascinating disorder.

REFERENCES

Albert-Stewart, P. L. (1986). Positive reinforcement in short-term treatment of an electively mute child: a case study. *Psychological Reports* 58:571–576.

American Psychiatric Association. (1987). *Diagnostic and Statistical Manual of Mental Disorders, Third Edition Revised (DSM-III-R)*. Washington, DC: American Psychiatric Association.

——— (1994). *Diagnostic and Statistical Manual of Mental Disorders, Fourth Edition (DSM-IV)*. Washington, DC: American Psychiatric Association.

Atlas, J. A. (1993). Symbol use in a case of elective mutism. *Perceptual and Motor Skills* 76:1079–1082.

Atoynatan, T. H. (1986). Elective mutism: involvement of the mother in the treatment of the child. *Child Psychiatry and Human Development* 17(1):15–27.

Baptiste, D. A., Jr. (1995). Therapy with a lesbian stepfamily with an electively mute child: a case report. *Journal of Family Psychotherapy* 6(1):1–20.

Black, B., and Uhde, T. W. (1992). Elective mutism as a variant of social phobia. *Journal of the Academy of Child and Adolescent Psychiatry* 31:1090–1094.

Boon, F. (1994). The selective mutism controversy. *Journal of the American Academy of Child and Adolescent Psychiatry* 33(2):283.

Bradley, S., and Sloman, L. (1975). Elective mutism in immigrant families. *Journal of the American Academy of Child Psychiatry* 14:510–514.

Brown, B., and Doll, B. (1988). Case illustration of classroom interventions with an elective mute child. *Special Services in the Schools* 5(1.5):107–125.

Browne, E., Wilson, V., and Laybourne, P. C. (1963). Diagnosis and treatment of elective mutism in children. *Journal of the Academy of Child Psychiatry* 2:605–617.

Carr, A., and Afnan, S. (1989). Concurrent individual and family therapy of elective mutism. *Journal of Family Therapy* 2:29–44.

Chethik, M. (1973). Amy: the intensive treatment of an elective mute. *Journal of the American Academy of Child Psychiatry* 12:482–498.

Clemente, J., Brafman, M., and Cohen, C. H. (1986). Concurrent treatment of mother and child in resolution of multigenerational separation and individuation difficulties. *Journal of Contemporary Psychotherapy* 16(2):140–150.

Croghan, L. M., and Craven, R. (1982). Elective mutism: learning from the analysis of a successful case history. *Journal of Pediatric Psychology* 7(1):85–93.

Crumley, F. E. (1990). The masquerade of mutism. *Journal of the American Academy of Child and Adolescent Psychiatry* 29(2):318:319.

——— (1993). Is elective mutism a social phobia? *Journal of the American Academy of Child and Adolescent Psychiatry* 32(5):1081–1082.

Fundudis, T., Kolvin, I., and Garside, R. F. (1979). *Speech Retarded and Deaf Children: Their Psychological Development*. London: Academic Press.

Jacobsen, T. (1995). Case study: Is selective mutism a manifestation of dissociative identity disorder? *Journal of the American Academy of Child and Adolescent Psychiatry* 34(7):863–866.

Kehle, T. J., Owen, S. V., and Cressy, E. T. (1990). The use of self-modeling as an intervention in school psychology: a case study of an elective mute. *School Psychology Review* 19(1):115–121.

Kolvin, I., and Fundudis, T. (1981). Elective mute children: psychological development and background factors. *Journal of Child Psychology and Psychiatry* 22(3):219–232.

Kussmaul, A. (1877). *Die Stoerungen der Sprache* [Language Disorders]. Leipzig: F. C. W. Vogel.

Lesser-Katz, M. (1986). Stranger reaction and elective mutism in young children. *American Journal of Orthopsychiatry* 56(3):458–469.

—— (1988). The treatment of elective mutism as stranger reaction. *Psychotherapy* 25(2):305–313.

Lindblad-Goldberg, M. (1986). Elective mutism in families with young children. *Family Therapy Collections* 18:31–42.

Lipton, H. (1980). Rapid reinstatement of speech using stimulus fading with a selectively mute child. *Journal of Behavior Therapy and Experimental Psychiatry* 11:147–149.

Marcus, A., Muller, F., Rothenberger, A., and Schmidt, M. H. (1993). Total mutism—a case report of a rare psychiatric disorder and approaches for behavior therapy. *Acta Paedopsychiatrica* 56:41–46.

Matson, J. L., Box, M. L., and Francis, K. L. (1992). Treatment of elective mute behavior in two developmentally delayed children using modeling and contingency management. *Journal of Behavior Therapy and Experimental Psychiatry* 23(3):221–229.

Nash, R. A., Thorpe, H. W., Andrews, M. M., and Davis, K. (1979). A management program for elective mutism. *Psychology in the Schools* 16(2):246–253.

Paniagua, F. A., and Saeed, M. A. (1987). Labeling and functional language in a case of psychological mutism. *Journal of Behavior Therapy and Experimental Psychiatry* 18:259–267.

—— (1988). A procedural distinction between elective and progressive mutism. *Journal of Behavior Therapy and Experimental Psychiatry* 19(3):207–210.

Piersel, W. C., and Kratochwill, T. R. (1981). A teacher-implemented contingency management package to assess and treat selective mutism. *Behavioral Assessment* 3:371–382.

Radford, P. (1977). A psychoanalytically-based therapy as the treatment of choice for a six-year-old elective mute. *Journal of Child Psychotherapy* 4(3):49–65.

Rasbury, W. C. (1974). Behavioral treatment of selective mutism: a case report. *Journal of Behavior Therapy and Experimental Psychiatry* 5:103–104.

Richards, C. S., and Hansen, M. K. (1978). A further demonstration of the efficacy of stimulus fading treatment of elective mutism. *Journal of Behavior Therapy and Experimental Psychiatry* 9:57–60.

Rosenberg, J. B., and Lindblad, M. B. (1978). Behavior therapy in a family context: treating elective mutism. *Family Process* 17:77–82.

Sanok, R. L., and Ascione, F. R. (1979). Behavioral interventions for childhood elective mutism: an evaluative review. *Child Behavior Therapy* 1(1):49–68.

Sanok, R. L., and Streifel, S. (1979). Elective mutism: generalization of verbal responding across people and settings. *Behavior Therapy* 10:357–371.

Scott, E. (1977). A desensitization programme for the treatment of mutism in a seven-year-old girl: a case report. *Journal of Child Psychology and Psychiatry* 18:263–270.

Sluckin, A., Foreman, N., and Herbert, M. (1991). Behavioral treatment programs and selectivity of speaking at follow-up in a sample of 25 selective mutes. *Australian Psychologist* 26(2):132–137.

Tramer, M. (1934). Elective Mutismus bei Kindern [Elective mutism in children]. *Zeitschrift fur Kinderpsychiatrie* 1:30–35.

Van Der Kooy, D., and Webster, C. D. (1975). A rapidly effective behavior modification program for an electively mute child. *Journal of Behavior Therapy and Experimental Psychiatry* 6:149–152.

Watson, T. S., and Kramer, J. J. (1992). Multimethod behavioral treatment of long-term selective mutism. *Psychology in the Schools* 29:359–366.

Williamson, D. A., Sewell, W. R., Sanders, S. H., et al. (1977). The treatment of reluctant speech using contingency management procedures. *Journal of Behavior Therapy and Experimental Psychiatry* 8:151–156.

Wright, H. H., and Cuccaro, M. L. (1994). Selective mutism continued. *Journal of the American Academy of Child and Adolescent Psychiatry* 33(4):593–594.

Wright, H. L., Jr. (1968). A clinical study of children who refuse to talk in school. *Journal of the American Academy of Psychiatry* 7:603–617.

PART I

ASSESSMENT AND TREATMENT PLANNING

2

PRACTICAL GUIDELINES FOR THE ASSESSMENT AND TREATMENT OF SELECTIVE MUTISM

Sara P. Dow, Barbara C. Sonies, Donna Scheib, Sharon E. Moss, and Henrietta L. Leonard

SELECTIVE MUTISM IS a disorder of childhood characterized by the total lack of speech in at least one specific situation (usually the classroom), despite the ability to speak in other situations. Recently there has been a shift in the etiological views on selective mutism, de-emphasizing psychodynamic factors and instead focusing on biologically mediated temperamental and anxiety components (Black and Uhde 1992, Crumley 1990, Golwyn and Weinstock 1990, Leonard and Topol 1993). Reports in the literature, in addition to our clinical work, suggest that selective mutism may be the manifestation of a shy, inhibited temperament most likely modulated by psychodynamic and psychosocial issues and in some cases associated with neuropsychological delays (developmental delays, speech and language disabilities, or difficulty processing social cues) (Figure 2–1). Although systematic study of this hypothesis is still needed, cognitive-behavioral treatment interventions, in addition to pharmacotherapy, have become more common than traditional psychodynamic approaches. This chapter provides practical guidelines for the assess-

ment and treatment of selective mutism based on our clinical experience along with reports from the literature.

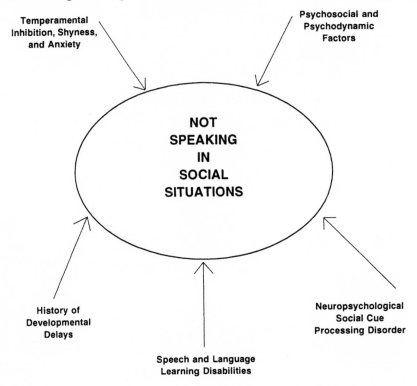

Figure 2–1. Factors that may influence speech and social inhibition

BACKGROUND

HISTORY AND DEFINITION

In the latter part of the 19th century, Kussmaul (1877) described a
disorder in which people would not speak in some situations, despite having the ability to speak. Kussmaul named this disorder
"aphasia voluntaria," thereby emphasizing what he thought was a

voluntary decision not to speak. When Tramer (1934) observed the same symptoms, he called the problem "elective mutism," with the belief that these children were "electing" not to speak. The most recent edition of the *Diagnostic and Statistic Manual of Mental Disorders (DSM-IV)* (American Psychiatric Association 1994) has adopted a new term: *selective mutism*. The change from "elective" to "selective" (implying that the children do not speak in "select" situations) is consistent with new theories of etiology that de-emphasize oppositional behavior and instead focus more on anxiety issues. The diagnosis of selective mutism, however, revolves around only one primary symptom: "consistent failure to speak in specific social situations . . . despite speaking in other situations" (American Psychiatric Association 1994, p. 115). Additional criteria require that the symptom last at least one month, be severe enough to interfere with educational or occupational achievement, and not be due to another problem (such as insufficient knowledge of the language, a communication disorder, pervasive developmental disorder, schizophrenia, or another psychotic disorder). Despite these criteria, the population of children with selective mutism remains heterogeneous, which could complicate treatment recommendations.

DIFFERENTIAL DIAGNOSIS

Since speech inhibition can be a secondary symptom of many other psychiatric disorders (including pervasive developmental disorder, schizophrenia, and severe mental retardation), differential diagnosis for selective mutism can be complex (American Psychiatric Association 1994). When a communication disorder is present, distinguishing between symptoms that are secondary to speech and language problems and those that are suggestive of selective mutism may be even more difficult. Although speech and language deficits can cause speech inhibition (Lerea and Ward 1965), several authors have reported that speech and language problems can also exist comorbidly with selective mutism (Kolvin and Fundudis 1981, Wilkins 1985, Wright 1968).

EPIDEMIOLOGY

Selective mutism has been described as a rare disorder, affecting fewer than 1 percent of school-age children, but little systematic research has been done to support this estimate. Using fairly strict diagnostic criteria, Fundudis and colleagues (1979) identified two selectively mute children in a survey of 3,300 seven-year-olds in Newcastle, U.K., a rate of 0.06 percent. In contrast, Brown and Lloyd (1975) reported a much higher prevalence of 0.69 percent (42/6,072 children). However, this estimate was obtained after only eight weeks of school, and fifty-six weeks later, the rate had fallen to 0.02 percent (1/6,072 children).

ETIOLOGY

Etiological explanations for selective mutism have varied widely (Leonard and Dow 1995). Some have explained it as a response to family neurosis, usually characterized by overprotective or domineering mothers and strict or remote fathers (Browne et al. 1963, Meijer 1979, Meyers 1984, Parker et al. 1960, Pustrom and Speers 1964). Others have suggested that the symptom could be a manifestation of unresolved psychodynamic conflict (Elson et al. 1965, Youngerman 1979). In addition, some have reported that it may develop as a reaction to trauma, such as sexual abuse or early hospitalization (MacGregor et al. 1994). Divorce, death of a loved one, and frequent moves have also been postulated to play a role in symptom development.

In the more recent literature, authors have noted a resemblance between selectively mute children and socially phobic adults (Black and Uhde 1992, Crumley 1990, Golwyn and Weinstock 1990, Leonard and Topol 1993). Crumley (1990) reported the case of a 29-year-old man who had been selectively mute at age 8½ years. The man remembered being afraid to speak for fear that he "might say or do the wrong thing" (Crumley 1990, p. 318). He also described experiencing "sudden episodes of intense anxiety" and physical symptoms that were suggestive of panic (shortness of breath, palpitations, dizziness) when he was placed in a situation where speech was expected. As an adult, the patient still had anxiety in social situations and often would not initiate conversation for fear that he would "say the wrong thing and embarrass myself" (Crumley 1990, p. 319). Crumley speculated that the patient's problems with social phobia might have been related to his initial elective (selective) mutism symptoms.

Black and Uhde (1992) described a selectively mute girl who had told her mother that she was reluctant to speak because "her voice sounded funny and she did not want others to hear it" (p. 1090). Her family psychiatric history was remarkable for paternal public-speaking anxiety and maternal childhood shyness. Boon (1994) reported the case of a 6-year-old girl who did not speak to adults. She explained her inability to speak by saying, "my brain wouldn't let me; my voice sounds strange" (p. 283). The girl's father was in treatment for panic disorder, and her paternal grandfather had had an anxiety disorder. Boon speculated that research on the pharmacotherapy of selective mutism "likely will support the view that elective mutism is an anxiety/OCD [obsessive-compulsive disorder] spectrum disorder" (p. 283).

PHENOMENOLOGY

Several authors found selective mutism to be more prevalent in females than males (Hayden 1980, Wergeland 1979, Wilkins 1985, Wright 1968). However, others found the disorder only slightly more frequent in females (Brown and Lloyd 1975, Kolvin and Fundudis 1981), and some found no sex difference (Parker et al. 1960). Onset is usually insidious, with parents reporting that the child "has always been this way" (Hayden 1980, Kolvin and Fundudis 1981, Leonard and Topol 1993, Wright 1968, Wright et al. 1985), but the diagnosis is often not made until the child enters kindergarten or first grade and verbal skills become more essential (5 to 6 years old).

Nearly all descriptions of selectively mute children in the literature have included some reference to their shyness, inhibition, or anxiety. Some have described them as "particularly sensitive, shy, afraid of everything strange or new" (Wergeland 1979, p. 219), others called them "unduly timid and sensitive" (Morris 1953, p. 667), and others reported "shy, timid, clinging behavior away from home" (Hayden 1980, p. 128). One author went so far as to characterize them as not only shy, but actually "socially inept" (Friedman and Karagan 1973, p. 250). Our clinical experience with selectively mute children has suggested that anxiety may play a much larger role than previously acknowledged, and these reports support such a hypothesis.

A wide variety of comorbid psychiatric problems have been described in children with selective mutism. Kolvin and Fundudis (1981) reported an increased incidence of elimination problems (as high as 42 percent for enuresis and 17 percent for encopresis, versus 15 percent and 2 percent for controls). Others found obsessive-compulsive features (Hayden 1980, Kolvin and Fundudis 1981, Wergeland 1979), school phobia (Elson et al. 1965, Parker et al. 1960, Pustrom and Speers 1964, Wright 1968), and depression (Wilkins 1985).

Although there have been no reports of systematic speech and language assessment, several authors have noted speech delays or problems among selectively mute children. Kolvin and Fundudis (1981) reported that the twenty-four selectively mute children in their study began speaking significantly later than 102 matched controls (27.3 months versus 21.9 months; no *p* value given). In addition, half (12/24) of these same selectively mute children had immaturities of speech at the time of evaluation, whereas only 9 percent (9/102) of the normal controls had any such problems. Wilkins (1985) reported that six (25 percent) of the twenty-four selectively mute children he studied had a delayed onset of speech and two (8.3 percent) had speech problems at the time of evaluation, while no such problems were found in any of the controls. Wright (1968) found articulation problems in five (21 percent) of his twenty-four patients, one of whom was dysarthric. Of note, these authors measured speech problems only and gave no reports of linguistic ability. Preliminary data from comprehensive speech and language assessments of selectively mute children evaluated in our clinic reveal that just less than one-half had mild to moderate expressive or receptive language delays severe enough to warrant intervention (unpublished data). It appears that the rate of speech and language delays in the selectively mute population (and the impact of such delays) merits further investigation.

ASSESSMENT

Any child who is being considered for a diagnosis of selective mutism should have a comprehensive evaluation to rule out other explanations for the mutism and to assess comorbid factors. An individualized treatment plan can then be developed.

PARENTAL INTERVIEW

Since most selectively mute children will not speak to clinicians, an interview with the parent or guardian of the child can provide essential information (Table 2-1).

A description of the child's symptom history, particularly onset (sudden or insidious), may help establish the diagnosis of selective mutism. Any patterns of behavior that are not characteristic of selective mutism, such as not talking to immediate family members, abrupt cessation of speech in one environment, or absence of speech in all settings, raise concerns about other neurological or psychiatric problems (e.g., autism, aphasia). A history of neurological insult, developmental delays, neuropsychological deficits, and/or atypical speech and language difficulties (such as problems with prosody) could be suggestive of Asperger's disorder, right hemisphere deficit disorder, or social emotional learning disabilities, rather than selective mutism (Voeller 1986, Weintraub and Mesulam 1983). Children with these disorders often have symptoms of shyness and social isolation and thus may appear similar to selectively mute children, but research suggests that their symptoms are based on an inability to process social cues.

Also of interest is the degree to which the child is verbally and nonverbally inhibited. Some selectively mute children are shy and anxious in unfamiliar environments, while others will interact in

Table 2–1.
Assessment of Selectively Mute Children

Areas	Parental Interview	Clinical Interview
Symptoms	• Type of onset (insidious, sudden) • Past treatments and efficacy • Where and to whom the child will speak	• Observations from interacting with the child
Social interaction	• Ability to make and keep friends • Extent and pattern of participation in social activities • Degree of shyness/ inhibition in familiar and foreign settings • Individuals to whom child will speak • Ability to communicate needs	• Observations of temperament made during interaction with child (shy? anxious? inhibited? interactive?)
Psychiatric	• Detailed assessment of psychiatric symptoms (use of a structured interview is preferred by some) • Family history of psychiatric problems and excessive shyness • Temperament during developmental stages	• Mental status examination
Medical	• Child's medical history, including illnesses or hospitalizations • Prenatal and perinatal history • Developmental history • Family medical history	• Physical examination, including screening for neurological or oral-sensorimotor problems

Table 2–1. Continued
Assessment of Selectively Mute Children

Areas	Parental Interview	Clinical Interview
Audiological	• Frequency of otitis media • Any reported concerns about hearing problems	• Peripheral sensitivity (pure-tone and speech stimuli) • Tympanometry and acoustic reflex (for middle ear)
Academic and cognitive	• Review of academic achievement (grades, teacher reports)	• Standardized tests of cognitive skills and achievement
Speech and language	• Reported complexity and fluency of child's speech at home • Nonverbal communication (gestures, etc.) • Any history of speech and language delays • Detailed description of child's speech production, language use, and comprehension • Discussion of environmental influences on language learning (bilingualism, etc.)	• Receptive language: assess using standardized tests • Expressive language: assess using audiotape and standardized testing, if possible (note lengh of utterances grammatical complexity, tone of voice) • Speech: assess using audiotape (note fluency, pronunciation, rhythm, stress, inflection, pitch, volume)

some way even if they will not speak (perhaps by nodding their head or smiling). Targeted questions about the child's verbal and nonverbal interaction, relationships with friends, and anxiety in social situations can be revealing. The child's social interaction outside of school, such as in a restaurant or on the telephone, should also be explored.

A structured diagnostic interview, such as the Diagnostic Interview for Children and Adolescents—Parent version (Herjanic and

Campbell 1977) or the Schedule for Affective Disorders and Schizophrenia for School-Age Children—Epidemiologic Version (Orvaschel
and Puig-Antich 1987) can be helpful for assessment of comorbid
psychiatric symptoms. Pervasive developmental disorder, schizophrenia, and mental retardation can cause speech inhibition and thus
might rule out a diagnosis of selective mutism.

Academic ability should also be discussed. Because it is difficult to evaluate children with selective mutism via traditional testing, minor learning disabilities may be overlooked. Parent and
teacher comments, academic reports, and standardized testing results
can all be helpful to evaluate the child's skills and determine whether
further testing is indicated.

Reviewing the child's medical history is essential because physical problems might underlie the child's mutism. Neurological injury
or delay can result in speech and language problems or social skills
deficits, both of which can exacerbate speech inhibition. In addition,
some authors have reported that early hospitalizations or abuse may
play a role in the development of selective mutism (MacGregor et
al. 1994). Hearing should also be checked (particularly if the child
has a history of frequent ear infections), since hearing problems are
sometimes associated with learning and language delays.

Family history of selective mutism, extreme shyness, or anxiety
disorders (social phobia, panic disorder, obsessive-compulsive disorder) may put the child at risk for developing similar problems and
should be thoroughly explored with the parents. In addition, a complete family history of any psychiatric or medical diagnoses, including response to treatment, can be helpful.

Evaluation of speech and language ability is essential. Factors
that might have influenced a child's language development, such as
a parent with identified speech and language problems, or a lack of
adequate exposure to the language (as in some bilingual homes),
should be considered. Inadequate or confusing language exposure
may result in expressive problems, and additional practice may be
necessary for the child to function at normal levels. Other questions
should focus on the child's ability to communicate his or her needs,

both verbally and nonverbally. Descriptions of the complexity and quality of language (mean length of utterance, range of vocabulary, use of difficult verb tenses and complicated grammar) can help one evaluate expressive language ability. Pragmatic language abilities, such as turn-taking in conversation, understanding of nonverbal communicative cues, and so on, should also be explored. Other questions might focus on the child's speech production (voice, fluency, resonance, rate, and rhythm), to identify phonological problems. It can also be helpful to have parents provide an audiotape of the child speaking at home (as detailed later), because few children with selective mutism will actually speak to clinicians.

Many checklists have been used to assess speech and language ability, including the Classroom Communication Checklist (Ripich and Spinelli 1985), the Interpersonal Language Skills Checklist (McConnell and Blagden 1986), and the Environmental Language Inventory (MacDonald 1978). We adapted these scales to create the National Institutes of Health Parent Checklist (Sonies et al. 1993; available upon request), which augments information provided by standardized speech and language testing. In this questionnaire, parents are asked to respond to statements regarding the expressive, receptive, and pragmatic abilities of their child, indicating frequency (never, rarely, sometimes, frequently, or always). This checklist, or others, can be used to supplement standardized speech and language testing.

CHILD ASSESSMENT

Interviewing the child is a crucial part of the assessment as it allows the clinician to directly observe the severity and nature of the child's mutism, as well as to pursue any concerns raised by the parents (Table 2-1).

Temperament, quality of interaction, and ability to communicate verbally and nonverbally can all be observed during the interview with the child. As most selectively mute children will not talk to the clinician, other forms of nonverbal communication (playing, drawing) may be used to assess anxiety or shyness in social situations. Some selectively mute children will avoid eye contact and withdraw from social situations, while others are more interactive and will smile, giggle, and nod answers to questions, even if they will not speak.

A review of the physical examination will ensure that the child has no medical problems that could potentially complicate the clinical picture. Oral sensory and motor ability should be evaluated, with particular note of any orofacial abnormalities that might interfere with articulation. Neurological difficulties, as evidenced by drooling, grimacing, muscular asymmetry, tongue and lip weakness, abnormal gag reflex, or impaired sucking or swallowing, can be relevant because they may impede the movements necessary for normal speech.

Auditory testing should be completed to ensure that hearing difficulties are not contributing to the mutism. Several studies have shown that even mild audiological impairments can have a negative effect on speech and language development (Fundudis et al. 1979). General tests of peripheral sensitivity (using both pure-tone and speech stimuli) are usually adequate to detect problems. In addition, tympanometry and acoustic reflex testing can be used to assess middle ear function.

Standardized psychological testing may be necessary to confirm parental and teacher reports of the child's cognitive abilities, particularly because many of these children are difficult to assess academically. While learning disabilities are rarely the cause of mutism, they could exacerbate the problem. Tests of intellectual capacity (which measure components of memory, attention, reasoning, and judgment) can be invaluable in obtaining a measure of the child's potential level of functioning. Many different tests are available, but the performance section of the Wechsler Intelligence Scale for Children–Revised (WISC-R) (Wechsler 1974) and Raven's Colored Progressive Matrices (Raven 1976) were found to be good measures of cognitive ability in our selective mutism clinic since children were not required to respond orally.

A formal speech and language evaluation, including components of receptive language, expressive language, and phonology, is an essential part of the assessment. While speech and language are closely tied, they are separate entities and thus require different types of assessment. Speech is "the activity of articulating speech sounds," while language involves higher cortical functioning: "the communication of thoughts by the use of meaningful units combined in a systematic way" (Bishop 1994, p. 556). A complete evaluation of the child's ability will utilize several different approaches, combining standardized testing with information obtained from the parents, as well as an audiotape of the child speaking at home.

Most of the children referred to our selective mutism clinic had never received formal speech and language testing, perhaps in part because of a misconception that nonverbal children cannot be evaluated for speech and language functioning. Several tests of receptive language ability that can be administered to nonverbal subjects are available. The Peabody Picture Vocabulary Test (Dunn and Dunn 1981) is useful as an initial screening for receptive language problems, since it can be administered nonverbally and it has been standardized for children as young as 2 years old. To evaluate more complex receptive ability, one could use a variety of other tests, including (but not limited to) the Token Test for Children (DiSimoni 1978), the Test for Auditory Comprehension of Language–Revised (Woolfolk 1985), the Test of Language Development (Hammil and Newcomer 1982), and the Detroit Test of Learning Aptitude–Primary (Hammil and Bryant 1986). For less responsive or immature children, the Utah Test of Language Development (Mecham and Jones 1989) or the Preschool Language Scale–3 (Zimmerman et al. 1991) might be more appropriate.

A prerecorded audiotape of the child speaking at home can be used to evaluate phonological ability, including length of utterances, grammatical construction, tone of voice, and response to verbalizations. In addition, one should be alert for any abnormalities of rhythm, stress, inflection, pitch, or volume. Speech defects have been noted to cause speech inhibition in some cases and thus could exacerbate the symptoms of selective mutism (Lerea and Ward 1965).

TREATMENT

Treatment for selective mutism has for a long time been considered difficult; some have described the disorder as intractable. Many different approaches have been used to treat this disorder, including a variety of behavioral techniques, psychodynamic approaches, family therapy, speech therapy, and most recently pharmacological intervention (for reviews, see Cline and Baldwin 1994, Kratochwill 1981, Tancer 1992). Unfortunately, the majority of treatment reports have been in case study format, many with only a single subject. While case studies may be helpful to describe a new approach or intervention, generalizing from such reports can be problematic. In many of these reports, procedures were not sufficiently described to allow for replication, outcome measures were not objective or standardized, alternative explanations for symptom remission were not explored, and unsuccessful cases were not reported (Wells 1987).

Some authors have attempted to increase validity using a more systematic case study approach, the "single-case experimental design" (Bauermeister and Jemail 1975, Cunningham et al. 1983). For example, objective symptom measures (such as number of words spoken per hour) have been used to quantify outcome, and treatment results have been compared to baseline. A few authors have even used multiple baselines (home, school, other settings). However, single-case experimental design is still limited by small sample size, and systematic trials with larger groups are needed. Only two controlled studies of treatment for selective mutism were found in the literature, one using behavioral therapy (Calhoun and Koenig 1973) and the other using pharmacotherapy with fluoxetine (Black and Uhde 1994). Both studies reported success in the treated group, as detailed below.

BEHAVIORAL

Behavioral interventions, based on principles of learning theory, have been the most frequently used treatment for selective mutism. Reed (1963) was one of the first to suggest that mutism could be a learned behavior and thus might respond to behavioral techniques such as reinforcement and stimulus fading. He hypothesized that mutism developed either as a means of getting attention or as an escape from anxiety. Treatment was thus directed at extinguishing all reinforcement for the mutism, while simultaneously bolstering self-confidence and decreasing anxiety.

There have been many subsequent attempts to use behavioral techniques to encourage speech in selectively mute children (the reader is referred to Cunningham et al. 1983, Labbe and Williamson 1984, and Sanok and Ascione 1979, for reviews). However, the only controlled study of behavioral therapy to date was that of Calhoun and Koenig (1973), which involved eight selectively mute children. In this study, children were randomly assigned to treatment or control groups, and data (number of words per 30 minutes) were collected by trained observers at baseline, posttreatment, and follow-up. Although treatment was not described in sufficient detail to assess or replicate, it appeared to consist of teacher and peer reinforcement of verbal behavior. Subjects who received active treatment were found to have significantly more vocalizations than untreated subjects five weeks after the start of treatment ($p < .01$), but improvement was not significant at follow-up one year later ($p < .10$).

In addition to this controlled study, there are numerous case reports of behavioral treatment for selective mutism. Most authors used some type of reinforcement for speaking, often combined with an absence of reinforcement for the mute behavior. Some also used punitive measures (forcing the child to sit in the corner, splashing the child with water), but these may have a tendency to increase a child's anxiety and thus would not be recommended. Stimulus fading, a technique similar to the desensitization used to treat social phobia, has also been reported to be an effective approach, particularly when combined with reinforcement (the reader is referred to Heimberg and Barlow 1991, for a review of cognitive-behavioral therapy for social phobia in adults). In stimulus fading, therapists set simple goals and then gradually increase the difficulty of the task. For example, Scott (1977) used this approach with a 7-year-old girl, gradually adding new people into a room in which the girl was speaking. Three months after the end of treatment, Scott reported that, although she "will always be a shy child and will possibly experience difficulty in communication . . . the problem of mutism no longer exists" (pp. 269–270).

Other authors have reported on the effectiveness of techniques such as shaping to initiate speech in the school setting (Austad et al. 1980). Shaping is a procedure in which the therapist reinforces mouth movements that approximate speech until true speech is achieved. Self-modeling, a technique in which the child watches videotaped segments of himself or herself performing desired behaviors (speaking, interacting), has also been tried with some success, though only with case studies (Dowrick and Hood 1978, Pigott and Gonzales 1987).

PSYCHODYNAMIC

While insight-oriented psychodynamic therapy was at one time the preferred treatment for selective mutism, cognitive-behavioral approaches are now being used with increasing frequency. Psychodynamic theory characterizes mutism as a manifestation of intrapsychic conflict, and treatment is focused on identifying and resolving such underlying conflicts. The treatment process can be time consuming, particularly if the child will not speak, and as a result many psychodynamic therapists have utilized art or play to facilitate communication and expedite therapy (Landgarten 1975).

FAMILY THERAPY

In older reports, family pathology was often postulated to be a causal factor in the development of selective mutism (Goll 1979, Lindblad-Goldberg 1986, Meijer 1979, Meyers 1984, Pustrom and Speers 1964). Authors described patterns of interaction in the family that seemed to encourage the child's mutism and thus prevent resolution of the symptom (Meyers 1984). Family therapy was used to identify and treat such dysfunctional patterns. Although no systematic research has been done using family therapy as the primary intervention for selective mutism, reports suggest that this approach can be effective in some cases (Goll 1979).

More recently, clinicians have not seen the child's symptom as a result of family pathology, but rather they have tried to involve family members in the design and implementation of a treatment plan. However, if family problems are identified that may be having an impact on the child's symptoms, a more traditional, insight-oriented family treatment approach could be appropriate.

PHARMACOTHERAPY

There are a few recent reports of pharmacological treatment for selective mutism, all using medications that have been helpful for social phobia (selective serotonin reuptake inhibitors). Golwyn and Weinstock (1990) described a 7-year-old girl with elective mutism and "associated shyness" who responded to phenelzine (up to 2 mg/day) with improvement noted as early as six weeks. She progressed from not speaking a word at school to being able to talk freely to teachers, peers, and therapists. Her father had panic disorder and had responded to phenelzine. Black and Uhde (1992) described a 12-year-old girl with elective mutism and social anxiety who responded to fluoxetine (20 mg/day); she was able to speak freely with adults and peers at school, and the response was maintained at seven months. Boon (1994) reported positive effects in the fluoxetine treatment of a 6-year-old selectively mute girl but did not provide details.

Black and Uhde (1994) recently completed a twelve-week trial of fluoxetine in children with elective mutism (placebo-controlled, parallel design). The six children taking active medication showed significant improvement on some ratings of mutism and anxiety but not on others, and subjects in both groups were still judged to be symptomatic at the conclusion of the study. Although interesting and somewhat promising, these results suggest that perhaps a longer trial, a more individualized dosage schedule, or combined intervention should be considered. In obsessive-compulsive disorder, a combination of pharmacotherapy and behavioral intervention is the treatment of choice (Leonard et al. 1994). Several investigators are currently studying the efficacy of serotonin reuptake inhibitors for the treatment of selective mutism, specifically fluoxetine and fluvoxamine. A medication trial should be considered if anxiety is a prominent factor or if symptoms have been resistant to other treatment attempts.

SPEECH THERAPY

Several authors have noted an increased prevalence of speech and language problems in the selectively mute population (Kolvin and Fundudis 1981, Wilkins 1985, Wright 1968). Smayling (1959) was the first to use speech therapy as the primary intervention for selective mutism, speculating that "speech defects, while not demonstrably the sole etiological factor, were causally related to the mutism" (p. 58). In Smayling's report, six selectively mute children who had some degree of speech or language disability were treated with half-hour sessions of speech therapy two to three times per week until the problems were resolved (two to twenty-one months). Therapists intentionally avoided mentioning the mutism or discussing the child's feelings, instead focusing on articulation and language training. Once the speech problems had been corrected, five of the six children began to speak in school. Strait (1958) also used speech therapy, but in conjunction with behavioral modification techniques such as reinforcement. Though both Smayling and Strait studied children with identified speech and language problems, it is likely that any selectively mute child could benefit from structured language practice.

SCHOOL-BASED MULTIDISCIPLINARY INDIVIDUALIZED TREATMENT PLAN

An effective individualized treatment program could be implemented in the school environment, with the coordinated efforts of parents, clinicians, and teachers. The goal of a treatment program should be to decrease the anxiety associated with speaking, while encouraging the child to interact and communicate (Table 2–2).

Table 2–2.
School-Based Multidisciplinary Intervention

Goals	Specific Interventions
Decrease anxiety	• Child should not be forced to speak • Keep child in regular classroom unless special needs other than selective mutism supersede • Less emphasis on verbal performance (play nonverbal games) • Encourage relationships with peers • Cognitive-behavioral interventions: desensitization with relaxation • Coordinate school-based program with out-of-school interventions (individual and family psychotherapy, pharmacotherapy)
Increase nonverbal communication	• Set up system for alternate means of communication (symbols, gestures, cards) • Small-group situations • Facilitate peer relationships
Increase social interaction	• Identify compatible peers for play in and out of school • Small-group situations • Activities that do not require verbal skills • Activities that encourage social skills
Increase verbal communication	• Structured behavioral modification plan: positive reinforcement for interactive and communicative behaviors, eventually reinforcement for speech • Speech and language therapy to develop linguistic skills • Pragmatically based language practice

Interventions that could be easily carried out by the classroom teacher include separating the class into small groups and identifying supportive peers. In some cases, an alternate means of communication (such as cards or gestures) might initially be necessary to allow the child to communicate basic needs. Any such system should be kept simple, however, so the child will still have incentive to communicate verbally.

Behavioral approaches can be helpful for encouraging the child to interact both verbally and nonverbally. At the start of a behavioral program, expectations should be kept low, perhaps rewarding the child for behaviors that he or she has already mastered or that are within reach. Once the child has gained confidence in his or her ability, the difficulty of the desired behavior can be increased. For example, one might begin by rewarding the child for whispering a single word and gradually increase the expectations until the child is saying the word in a normal volume. The type of reward could also be chosen according to the child's preferences (favorite candy, social praise, etc.). Once the child has become comfortable speaking in one environment, attempts can be made to generalize speech to other individuals or environments, using techniques such as stimulus fading.

The assistance of a speech therapist could be helpful in the development of a behavioral program for selective mutism, even if no specific speech and language impairments have been identified. Some selectively mute children have reported that they are afraid they will say the wrong thing or that their voice sounds funny, and speech and language practice could help such children gain confidence in their linguistic ability. Treatment might focus on perfecting pronunciation skills, increasing comprehension, and learning pragmatic skills, such as turn-taking during conversation. Practicing real-life interchanges until they have become automatic and less stressful might eventually help reduce a child's social inhibitedness.

SUMMARY

This chapter is a response to questions raised by families, clinicians, and educators in the course of evaluating selectively mute children in our clinic. Although ongoing studies of phenomenology and treatment were not yet completed, it was thought that there was an urgent need for practical information regarding assessment and treatment. Teachers and parents had asked how to treat these children and had questioned the appropriateness of special educational placements, yet no literature was available to assist them and many of the clinicians they turned to were unfamiliar with this disorder.

In our opinion, any child referred for selective mutism deserves a comprehensive assessment that addresses neurological, psychiatric, audiological, social, academic, and speech and language concerns. In the past, many of these children have not received complete assessments, either because clinicians believed they were untestable due to lack of verbal response or because clinicians deemed such assessments unnecessary. Our experience has been that it is not only possible to evaluate these children, but it is essential. Such evaluations can play an important role in identifying primary and comorbid issues and in developing appropriate treatment. Cognitive-behavioral, psychodynamic, pharmacological, and speech and language treatment approaches could all be integrated to decrease anxiety and to encourage speech and social interaction. Further systematic research will be required to evaluate the comparative effectiveness of these approaches.

REFERENCES

American Psychiatric Association. (1994). *Diagnostic and Statistical Manual of Mental Disorders, Fourth Edition (DSM-IV)*. Washington, DC: American Psychiatric Association.

Austad, L. S., Sinninger, R., and Stricken, A. (1980). Successful treatment of a case of elective mutism. *Behavior Therapist* 3:18–19.

Bauermeister, J. J., and Jemail, J. A. (1975). Modification of "elective mutism" in the classroom setting: a case study. *Behavior Therapy* 6:246–250.

Bishop, D. V. M. (1994). Developmental disorders of speech and language. In *Child and Adolescent Psychiatry: Modern Approaches*, ed. M. Rutter, E. Taylor, and L. Hersov, pp. 546–568. Oxford, England: Blackwell Scientific.

Black, B., and Uhde, T. W. (1992). Elective mutism as a variant of social phobia. *Journal of the American Academy of Child and Adolescent Psychiatry* 31:1090–1094.

———— (1994). Fluoxetine treatment of elective mutism: a double-blind, placebo-controlled study. *Journal of the American Academy of Child and Adolescent Psychiatry* 33:1000–1006.

Boon, E. (1994). The selective mutism controversy. *Journal of the American Academy of Child and Adolescent Psychiatry* 33:283.

Brown, J. B., and Lloyd, H. (1975). A controlled study of children not speaking at school. *Journal of the Association of Workers for Maladjusted Children* 3:49–63.

Browne, E., Wilson, V., and Laybourne, P. C. (1963). Diagnosis and treatment of elective mutism in children. *Journal of the American Academy of Child Psychiatry* 2:605–617.

Calhoun, J., and Koenig, K. P. (1973). Classroom modification of elective mutism. *Behavior Therapy* 4:700–702.

Cline, T., and Baldwin, S. (1994). *Selective Mutism*. London: Whurr.

Crumley, F. E. (1990). The masquerade of mutism. *Journal of the American Academy of Child and Adolescent Psychiatry* 29:318–319.

Cunningham, C. E., Cataldo, M. F., Mallion, C., et al. (1983). A review and controlled single case evaluation of behavioral approaches to the management of elective mutism. *Child and Family Behavioral Therapy* 5:25–49.

DiSimoni, F. (1978). *The Token Test for Children*. Boston: Teaching Resources.

Dowrick, P. W., and Hood, M. (1978). Transfer of talking behaviours across settings using faked films. In *New Zealand Conference for Research in Applied Behavioural Analysis*, ed. E. L. Glynn and S. S. McNaughton. Auckland, NZ: University of Auckland Press.

Dunn, L. M., and Dunn, L. M. (1981). *Peabody Picture Vocabulary Test-Revised*. Circle Pines, MN: American Guidance Services.

Elson, A., Pearson, C., Jones, C. D., and Schumacher, E. (1965). Follow up study of childhood elective mutism. *Archives of General Psychiatry* 13:182–187.

Friedman, R., and Karagan, N. (1973). Characteristics and management of elective mutism in children. *Psychology in the Schools* 10:249–254.

Fundudis, T., Kolvin, I., and Garside, R. (1979). *Speech Retarded and Deaf Children: Their Psychological Development*. London: Academic Press.

Goll, K. (1979). Role structure and subculture in families of elective mute children. *Family Process* 18:55–68.

Golwyn, D. H., and Weinstock, R. C. (1990). Phenelzine treatment of elective mutism: a case report. *Journal of Clinical Psychiatry* 51:384–385.

Hammil, D. D., and Bryant, B. R. (1986). *The Detroit Test of Learning Aptitude–Primary*. Austin, TX: Pro-ED.

Hammil, D. D., and Newcomer, P. L. (1982). *The Test of Language Development*. Austin, TX: Pro-ED.

Hayden, T. L. (1980). Classification of elective mutism. *Journal of the American Academy of Child Psychiatry* 19:118–133.

Heimberg, R. G., and Barlow, D. H. (1991). New developments in cognitive-behavioral therapy for social phobia. *Journal of Clinical Psychiatry* 5211(suppl):21–30.

Herjanic, B., and Campbell, W. (1977). Differentiating psychiatrically disturbed children on the basis of a structured psychiatric interview. *Journal of Abnormal Child Psychology* 5:127–135.

Kolvin, I., and Fundudis, T. (1981). Elective mute children: psychological, development, and background factors. *Journal of Child Psychology and Psychiatry* 22:219–232.

Kratochwill, T. R. (1981). *Selective Mutism: Implications for Research and Treatment*. Hillsdale, NJ: Erlbaum.

Kussmaul, A. (1877). *Die Storungen der Sprache*. Leipzig: F. C. W. Vogel.

Labbe, E. E., and Williamson, D. A. (1984). Behavioral treatment of elective mutism: a review of the literature. *Clinical Psychology Review* 4:273–294.

Landgarten, H. (1975). Art therapy as a primary mode of treatment for an elective mute. *American Journal of Art Therapy* 14:121–125.

Leonard, H. L., and Dow, S. P. (1995). Selective mutism. In *Anxiety Disorders in Children and Adolescents*, ed. J. March, pp. 235–250. New York: Guilford.

Leonard, H. L., Swedo, S. E., Allen, A. J., and Rapoport, J. L. (1994). Obsessive-compulsive disorder. In *International Handbook of Phobic and Anxiety Disorders in Children and Adolescents*, ed. T. H. Ollendick, N. J. King, and W. Yule, pp. 207–221. New York: Plenum.

Leonard, H. L., and Topol, D. A. (1993). Elective mutism. *Child and Adolescent Psychiatry Clinics of North America* 2:695–707.

Lerea, L., and Ward, B. (1965). Speech avoidance among children with oral-communication defects. *Journal of Psychology* 60:265–270.

Lindblad-Goldberg, M. (1986). Elective mutism in families with young children. In *Treating Young Children in Family Therapy*, vol. 18, ed. L. Combrinck Graham, pp. 31–42. Rockville, MD: Aspen.

MacDonald, J. (1978). *Environmental Language Inventory*. San Antonio, TX: Psychological Corporation.

MacGregor, R., Pullar, A., and Cundall, D. (1994). Silent at school: elective mutism and abuse. *Archives of Diseases of Childhood* 70:540–541.

McConnell, N., and Blagden, C. (1986). *Interpersonal Language Skills Checklist*. East Moline, IL: LinguiSystems.

Mecham, M. J., and Jones, J. D. (1989). *The Utah Test of Language Development-3*. Austin, TX: Pro-ED.

Meijer, A. (1979). Elective mutism in children. *Israeli Annals of Psychiatry and Related Disciplines* 17:93–100.

Meyers, S. V. (1984). Elective mutism in children: a family systems approach. *American Journal of Family Therapy* 22(4):39–45.

Morris, J. V. (1953). Cases of elective mutism. *American Journal of Mental Deficiency* 57:661–668.

Orvaschel, H., and Puig-Antich, J. (1987). *Schedule for Affective Disorders and Schizophrenia for School-Age Children: Epidemiologic Version*. Medical College of Pennsylvania, Eastern Pennsylvania Psychiatric Institute.

Parker, E. B., Olsen, T. F., and Throckmorton, M. C. (1960). Social case work with elementary school children who do not talk in school. *Social Work* 5:64–70.

Pigott, H. E., and Gonzales, F. P. (1987). Efficacy of video tape self-modeling in treating an electively mute child. *Journal of Clinical Child Psychology* 16:106–110.

Pustrom, E., and Speers, R. W. (1964). Elective mutism in children. *Journal of the American Academy of Child Psychiatry* 3:287–297.

Raven, J. C. (1976). *The Colored Progressive Matrices*. London: H. K. Lewis.

Reed, G. (1963). Elective mutism in children: a reappraisal. *Journal of Child Psychology and Psychiatry* 4:99.

Ripich, D., and Spinelli, F. M. (1985). Classroom Communication

Checklist. In *School Discourse Strategies*, ed. D. Ripich and F. M. Spinelli. San Diego: College Hill.

Sanok, R. L., and Ascione, F. R. (1979). Behavioral interventions for elective mutism: an evaluative review. *Child Behavior Therapy* 1:49–67.

Scott, E. (1977). A desensitisation programme for the treatment of mutism in a seven year old girl: a case report. *Journal of Child Psychology and Psychiatry* 18:263–270.

Smayling, J. M. (1959). Analysis of six cases of voluntary mutism. *Journal of Speech and Hearing Disorders* 24:55–58.

Sonies, B. C., Scheib, D., and Moss, S. (1993). *National Institutes of Health Parent Checklist*. Bethesda, MD: National Institutes of Health.

Strait, R. (1958). A child who was speechless in school and social life. *Journal of Speech and Hearing Disorders* 23:253–254.

Tancer, N. K. (1992). Elective mutism. In *Advances in Clinical Child Psychology*, vol. 14, ed. B. B. Lahey and A. E. Kazdin, pp. 265–288. New York: Plenum.

Tramer, M. (1934). Elektiver Mutismus bei Kindern. *Zeitschrift Fur Kinderpsychiatrie* 1:30–35.

Voeller, K. (1986). Right-hemisphere deficit syndrome in children. *American Journal of Psychiatry* 143:1004–1009.

Wechsler, D. (1974). *Manual for the Wechsler Intelligence Scale for Children–Revised*. New York: Psychological Corporation.

Weintraub, S., and Mesulam, M. (1983). Developmental learning disabilities and the right hemisphere. *Archives of Neurology* 40:463–468.

Wells, K. (1987). Scientific issues in the conduct of case studies: annotation. *Journal of Child Psychology and Psychiatry* 28:783–790.

Wergeland, H. (1979). Elective mutism. *Acta Psychiatrica Scandinavica* 59:218–228.

Wilkins, R. (1985). A comparison of elective mutism and emotional disorders in children. *British Journal of Psychiatry* 146:198–203.

Woolfolk, E. C. (1985). *The Test for Auditory Comprehension of Language–Revised*. Allen, TX: DLM Teaching Resources.

Wright, H. H., Miller, M. D., Cook, M. A., and Littman, J. R. (1985). Early identification and intervention with children who refuse to speak. *Journal of the American Academy of Child Psychiatry* 24:739–746.

Wright, H. L. (1968). A clinical study of children who refuse to talk in school. *Journal of the American Academy of Child Psychiatry* 7:603–617.

Youngerman, J. (1979). The syntax of silence: electively mute therapy. *International Review of Psychoanalysis* 6:283–295.

Zimmerman, I. L., Steiner, V. G., and Pond, R. E. (1991). *The Preschool Language Scale-3*. New York: Psychological Corporation.

3

WHEN TO INTERVENE IN SELECTIVE MUTISM: THE MULTIMODAL TREATMENT OF A CASE OF PERSISTENT SELECTIVE MUTISM

Shawn Powell and Mahlon Dalley

SELECTIVE MUTISM OCCURS in less than 1 percent of all mental health referrals and has been described as a rare, disabling condition (American Psychiatric Association 1994, Golwyn and Weinstock 1990). As a disorder, selective mutism describes the behavior of children who generally have normal language development yet only talk to a small group of relatives and peers (Friedman and Karagan 1973, Griffith et al. 1975, Kratochwill 1981, Porjes 1992, Silver 1985). The average age of diagnosis for selective mutism is 5 to 7 years old, and the disorder usually occurs when a child initially enters school and refuses to talk to classmates, teachers, or strangers (Black and Uhde 1992, Cunningham et al. 1983, Klin and Volkmar 1993, Krohn et al. 1992).

According to the *Diagnostic and Statistical Manual of Mental Disorders–Fourth Edition* (APA 1994), the primary feature of selective mutism is the "persistent failure to speak in specific social situations . . ." (p. 114). Compared to other childhood disorders, the sex ratio for selective mutism is unusual in that it occurs more often in females than in males (Silver 1985, Tancer 1992). Selective mutism is normally accompanied by other problematic behaviors (Cunningham et al. 1983, Kratochwill 1981, Rutter 1977). Tancer (1992) states, "Elective mutism has been defined very broadly so that children with diverse psychopathology are grouped together" (p. 265). Children manifesting selective mutism have been described as shy, timid, anxious, socially withdrawn, oppositional, controlling, having unpleasant temperaments, and being poor school performers (Atlas 1993, Black and Uhde 1992, Krohn et al. 1992, Tancer 1992).

Children exhibiting selective mutism tend to look normal and are not usually impacted by the presence of physical or mental defects that would contribute to their refusal to talk (Nash et al. 1979). Lumb and Wolff (1988) indicated that children with selective mutism, regardless of their silent behavior, appear capable of learning and typically use their skills in normal ways, with the exception of talking. Most children displaying this disorder communicate nonverbally using signs or gestures, and most talk to their parents (Cunningham et al. 1983).

Brown and Lloyd (1975) in a study of 6,072 children entering kindergarten indicated that 42 (0.7%) were not speaking 8 weeks after kindergarten started, although they talked in other environments. A 12-month follow-up study found that over 90% of the 42 students originally not talking in school were speaking. In reflecting on the causes of selective mutism, Brown and Lloyd considered that the behaviors that constitute this condition are likely an adaptation reaction. In reviewing Brown and Lloyd's work, Tancer (1992) agreed that selective mutism in children initially attending school could be transient and may represent normal separation anxiety or an adjustment disorder, with the implication that time and normal development would allow for the emergence of speech. Wilkens (1985) distinguished transient selective mutism from persistent selective mutism. The present study further differentiated transient selective mutism as occurring infrequently in children generally under the age of 5, lasting less than 6 months, and typically displayed in one environment. Persistent selective mutism was defined as occurring chronically in children over the age of 5, for more than 6 months, and typically displayed in more than one environment.

In treating selective mutism, a concerted effort must be undertaken to determine whether interventions are actually necessary. Lumb and Wolff (1988) pointed out that the majority of studies they reviewed did not consider justifications for interventions as factors in treatment planning. It seems that the majority of children exhibiting selective mutism are subjected to various treatment modalities because their behaviors are difficult to understand and frustrate adults. In deciding whether treatment is warranted, the impact of selective mutism on childhood developmental factors has to be reviewed (i.e., social adjustment and the inability to interact fully in various aspects of home or school).

The nonverbal behaviors involved in selective mutism have been linked to anxiety and fear and have been viewed as a developmental variant of social phobia (Black and Uhde 1992, Cunningham et al. 1983, Friedman and Karagan 1973, Shreeve 1991). Conversely, selective mutism has been perceived as a desire to control others (Kratochwill et al. 1979, Krohn et al. 1992). Some authors have also viewed selective mutism's etiology as the result of the desire to control others and the desire to control anxiety (Kratochwill 1981, Krohn et al. 1992, Silver 1985). Refusing to speak in a given or selected environment has also been perceived as a natural behavior (Lumb and Wolff 1988).

Numerous authors have viewed selective mutism as learned behavior (Albert-Stewart 1986, Cliffe 1991, Kehle et al. 1990, Kratochwill 1981, Porjes 1992, Reed and Mees 1967, Watson and Kramer 1992). Friedman and Karagan (1973) reported that learning theorists view nonverbal behavior as a learned response in which the refusal to speak is a method of manipulating the environment. The treatment of selective mutism appears to be best facilitated by combining various behavioral techniques (e.g., positive reinforcement, shaping, desensitization, modeling, extinction, etc.) (Kratochwill 1981, Matson et al. 1992, Watson and Kramer 1992).

Treatment modalities using forced approaches to making a child speak usually have high failure rates (Friedman and Karagan 1973). Watson and Kramer (1992) indicated that greater gains are made in resolving selective mutism when nonverbal behaviors are extinguished and verbal behaviors are reinforced, rather than when only verbal behaviors are reinforced. When acceptable levels of speech have been achieved, Cunningham et al. (1983) indicated that positive reinforcement can improve speech generalization.

Other researchers have incorporated treatment interventions outside strict behavioral approaches in treating selective mutism (Afnan and Carr 1989, Atoynatan 1986, Wright et al. 1985). Such interventions have often included a combination of family therapy and behavioral treatments. In two successful case studies, reinforcements were given by parents at school, with family praise and encouragement provided at home (Krohn et al. 1992, Nash et al. 1979). Group therapy has also been used to treat selective mutism. Bozigar and Hansen (1984) treated four female children with selective mutism in a mental health center using group therapy. Relaxation and deep breathing techniques were found to facilitate speech generalization in their treatment interventions. The importance of cooperating with the children's schools in order to generalize positive treatment gains was emphasized. Bozigar and Hansen reported the successful treatment of three children in their group and indicated failure to maintain close liaisons with the school as the reason for treatment failure in the fourth case.

Barlow and colleagues (1986) perceived play therapy as a "nonverbal solution to a nonverbal problem" (p. 49), and employed sibling play therapy, individual play therapy, and family consultation in their successful treatment of a case of selective mutism. Play therapy was used to create an intimate setting through which the child with selective mutism modeled behavioral changes in a nonthreatening environment.

In reviewing the literature on selective mutism, Wright and colleagues (1994) reported that only two case studies describe administering medication for its treatment. In treating a 12-year-old girl who had not spoken in school for five years, Black and Uhde (1992) administered a trial of desipramine with minimal success and then switched to a trial of fluoxetine. The second medication successfully treated the selective mutism. A seven-month follow-up indicated that the child was talking normally. Golwyn and Weinstock (1990) administered a sixteen-week trial of phenelzine in treating a child displaying selective mutism with associated shyness. A five-month follow-up indicated that the child was talking normally.

Porjes (1992) developed a four-stage learning theory approach for the treatment of two subjects with selective mutism. These four stages included: (1) ecological analysis implemented with the understanding that the child's nonverbal behaviors are adaptive and functional, not pathological; (2) development of reinforcement lists compiled with input from the child's teachers and parents; (3) elicitation of initial speech employing behavioral management techniques; and (4) generalization of speech to new situations and people (e.g., talking on the telephone, talking in the regular classroom after school, and involving other adults and students in the school).

IDENTIFICATION AND TREATMENT MODEL

The identification and treatment of selective mutism involves numerous considerations. As in any childhood disorder, these considerations include the development factors responsible for the remediation of symptoms when little or no intervention occurs. However, postponing diagnosis and treatment by waiting until symptoms escalate can greatly affect a child's behavior and development. To this end, a four-step identification and treatment model for selective mutism is proposed.

This model's first step involves considering the length of time the selective mutism has been present, the child's age, the consistency of the disorder, and the impact the selective mutism has on the child. These issues are important in determining whether the child's behavior suggests further involvement, or whether developmentally the selective mutism will most likely dissipate without treatment.

Step 1. Determining if selective mutism is present:

  a. Length of time selective mutism has occurred
  b. Age of child
  c. Consistency of selective mutism in multiple settings
  d. Impact of selective mutism on child

Step 2. Determining if selective mutism is transient or persistent

Transient selective mutism	Persistent selective mutism
a. Child is 5 or younger	a. Child is older than 5
b. Selective mutism has existed less than 6 months	b. Selective mutism has existed longer than 6 months
c. Selective mutism has existed intermittently	c. Selective mutism has existed consistently
d. Selective mutism exists in one environment	d. Selective mutism exists in more than one environment
If **transient**, monitor and if needed refer to step 3.	If **persistent**, apply steps 3 and 4.

Step 3. Evaluations

  a. Medical
  b. Speech and Language
  c. Psychological evaluation including:
    1. Intellectual assessment
    2. Emotional and behavioral assessment
    3. Observations in home and school
    4. Family/parent/teacher interviews

Step 4. Treatment/intervention

  a. Explaining selective mutism to family, parents, and teachers
  b. Use of Porjes's (1992) four-stage learning theory treatment model
  c. Use of other interventions as appropriate
    1. Family conferences/counseling
    2. Parental involvement in treatment
    3. Parent/teacher/psychologist conferences
    4. Play therapy

**Figure 3–1. Identification and treatment
of selective mutism**

Silver (1985) reported that studies of selective mutism seldom distinguish between transient and persistent selective mutism. In response, the model's second step determines whether the child is manifesting transient or persistent selective mutism. If the child displays transient selective mutism, the recommended course of action is to monitor the child to allow for the spontaneous remission of the disorder. Because of its association with anxiety, psychologists involved with children displaying selective mutism need to ascertain whether the presented disorder represents persistent selective mutism or is the result of another factor such as separation anxiety. If the child is entering kindergarten or first grade and the selective mutism has existed consistently for longer than six months in multiple environments, this suggests persistent selective mutism. In this case, evaluations and intervention measures are recommended.

If persistent selective mutism is presented, the third step of this model details specific evaluations and the order in which they are best administered. If medical examinations do not discern a physical reason for the disorder, and speech and language evaluations indicate normal speech (i.e., evaluating language samples from recordings of the child talking to a parent), then psychological evaluation is recommended. This evaluation should include an intellectual assessment to rule out the presence of developmental delays, an emotional and behavioral assessment to rule out emotional disabilities, home and school observations, and interviews with the family, parents, and teachers to determine the impact of the persistent selective mutism on the child.

The model's fourth step presents treatment and intervention strategies for remediating persistent selective mutism. Explaining what selective mutism is to the adults involved with the child is the first part of this treatment design. This educational component gives everyone working with the child a common understanding of the child's behavior so they can better assist in the child's treatment. Porjes's (1992) four-stage learning theory model for the treatment of selective mutism is highlighted as a particularly efficacious treatment strategy. The use of other interventions designed to improve the child's communications as deemed appropriate is recommended (e.g., family/parent/teacher involvement, play therapy, etc.).

CASE STUDY

The child in this study was a 6-year-old girl enrolled in a public kindergarten class. She attended public school on a half-day basis in the afternoon and lived with her natural parents and 3-year-old sister. The child attended a day-care program eight months before entering public school. She reportedly stopped talking to people other than her immediate family when she started the day-care program. After the child had been in kindergarten two months, the child's teacher referred her to the school's intervention team with the stated concern, "Does not talk to anyone except immediate family." Thus, the child had not spoken in an educational setting for ten months prior to school-based evaluations and treatment. It was also indicated that the child displayed selective mutism in other environments, for example, her peers' homes, restaurants, and so on. This suggested that her condition represented persistent selective mutism.

The child's age, extended time, consistency, and the multiple environments in which selective mutism had been displayed were considered in determining whether treatment was warranted. Another treatment consideration was the impact that not speaking in school was having on the child's social interactions and development. Although she was actively involved with school activities and clearly learning, she was not fully participating in all aspects of her classroom (e.g., plays, songs, and oral responses). Therefore, the inhibiting nature of the disorder was considered in deciding if treatment should be undertaken. The child's own desire to speak in school was an important factor dictating the need for treatment. Prior to and during treatment, she repeatedly informed her parents that she wanted to talk in school.

ASSESSMENT

The child was first administered a pediatric medical examination. The medical results did not indicate the presence of physical disorders that would have contributed to selective mutism. A 20-minute recording of the child speaking to her mother at home was then evaluated by a speech pathologist. The speech pathologist's evaluation did not discern any difficulties existing in the child's speech or language abilities.

Following the medical examination and speech and language evaluation, the child was then assessed by a school psychologist before treatment interventions began. Prior to the examinations and evaluations conducted in reference to her manifested selective mutism, the child had not been evaluated or received treatment for any condition other than routine medical examinations. Klin and Volkmar (1993) indicated that in the presence of selective mutism other comorbid factors such as mental deficiencies need to be considered and ruled out when possible. Therefore, the following assessment procedures were utilized: Test of Non Verbal Intelligence-2, Peabody Picture Vocabulary Test–Revised, Bender Visual Motor Gestalt Test, Burks' Behavioral Rating Scale, Walker Problem Behavior Identification Checklist, figure drawings, classroom observations, and family/parent/teacher interviews.

The child's nonverbal mental abilities were in the average range, while her receptive vocabulary scores fell in the low average range. Her visual motor developmental age equaled a percentile ranking of 60. This evaluation of the child's mental abilities ruled out the presence of developmental delays or mental deficiencies contributing to selective mutism.

Indications of treatment effectiveness relative to the child's manifested behaviors at school and home were gathered through pre- and posttreatment ratings. The referring classroom teacher and both of the child's parents completed behavioral rating scales independently. On the pretreatment scales, in addition to the observable selective mutism, all three raters indicated that the child's manifested immaturity existed above the problematic level as measured by the Walker Problem Behavior Identification Checklist. The child's average t score as determined by the three raters was 70. The child's teacher and mother rated her withdrawal in the significant range on the Burks' Behavioral Rating Scale. When observed in class, the child was attentive and actively participated in the class's activities. She responded to questions concerning shapes and colors accurately by pointing to objects the teacher asked about (e.g., a triangle, a square, or an object whose color she was asked to identify). Her responses were equivalent to those of the other students in the class, with the exception that they were communicated nonverbally.

TREATMENT

As advocated by Paniagua and Saeed (1988), interventions focused on improving the child's verbal interactions with others and did not become enmeshed with the condition's etiology. Treatment programming was designed according to Barlow et al.'s (1986) guidance that interventions be applied in a manner consistent with the child's comfort level. The four-stage learning theory treatment approach developed by Porjes (1992) was used as an intervention guide. Treatment was conducted over a six-month period, with a six-month follow-up completed after the child had entered first grade.

The first stage of Porjes's (1992) approach to treating selective mutism, an ecological analysis, was accomplished prior to intervention. An assessment of the child and her family was conducted cojointly by the school psychologist and school nurse. This assessment of the family's communication behaviors revealed that the child whispered to her mother in response to verbal questions asked by strangers. This behavior was modified as the child's mother was asked not to act as an "interpreter" for the child. The family's communications were further modified by asking family members to make the child respond verbally for herself, and to give her positive verbal reinforcement when she talked in environments where she had displayed selective mutism. This approach applied Watson and Kramer's (1992) suggestion that greater treatment gains are made in resolving selective mutism when nonverbal behaviors are extinguished and verbal behaviors are reinforced, rather than when verbal behaviors only are reinforced.

In keeping with Porjes's (1992) second treatment stage, developing reinforcement lists, a positive reinforcement list was compiled by the child's mother and classroom teacher. The rewards selected were verbal praise (e.g., "It's good to hear you talking," "Good job"), individual time with her mother, and material rewards consisting of small toys or candy.

BEHAVIORAL TECHNIQUES

Porjes's (1992) third stage, eliciting speech through behavioral interventions, was then employed by having the child's mother talk with her in her classroom after school. In this manner the child was exposed to shaping, positive reinforcement, and desensitization. These three behavioral techniques were used in combination to elicit speech from the child in her classroom, which was an environment where she had previously been silent.

During the first three sessions, when the child talked to her mother in her classroom after school, she was given a material reward by her teacher. After the third session, the material rewards were replaced by verbal praise and being able to spend time alone with her mother. These rewards were initially given on a continuous reinforcement one-to-one ratio—every time the child spoke in the classroom she was verbally reinforced. As she began talking to her mother spontaneously, the reinforcements were shifted to an intermittent ratio schedule.

This specific after-school intervention occurred sixteen times. During the first eight sessions, if anyone entered the classroom while the child was talking with her mother, she became silent. From the ninth to last session of this intervention, the child talked to her mother when others entered the classroom. When this occurred, she was immediately given positive verbal reinforcement by the individuals who had entered the classroom.

The child was audio-recorded in an interview conducted by her mother in the classroom. The teacher's voice, asking the same questions the child's mother had asked, was then dubbed over the child's mother's voice on the tape. The result was an audio tape that featured the teacher "asking" the child a series of questions to which she "responded." This audio tape was played in the classroom with the child, her mother, teacher, and school psychologist present. This intervention was designed to allow the child to hear herself respond to her teacher, and thus use her own voice as a model. During the playback of this audio tape the child manifested signs of anxiety, shaking hands, blinking, and looking around the room. After listening to the tape, she was verbally reinforced by all the adults present. Because this intervention was believed to have increased the child's anxiety, it was not used again as advised by Barlow et al. (1986).

Six weeks following the start of treatment the child had not spoken to anyone at school other than her mother. At this point, play therapy with the school psychologist was applied in addition to the after-school sessions taking place with the child's mother. The play therapy sessions followed Axline's (1947) nondirected treatment combined with verbal positive reinforcement given on an intermittent basis when the child spoke. Eighteen play therapy sessions, each lasting 30 minutes, were conducted during the remainder of the treatment regime on a weekly basis over a five-month period.

SPEECH GENERALIZATION

Approximately four weeks following the introduction of play therapy and while the after-school sessions with her mother were still ongoing, the child spoke to her teacher after school. This occurred one year to the week after she had been enrolled in the day-care program where the selective mutism had first been displayed. After the child talked to her teacher, she became self-directed and started verbalizing during play therapy sessions. This verbalization included self-talk and self-initiated conversations. As she started talking, speech modeling through role plays and conversations were incorporated into the play therapy to further encourage her to speak at school.

In keeping with Porjes's (1992) fourth treatment stage, generalization of speech to new situations and people, the child was involved in speaking to other adults and students at the school on a gradual basis. This gradual introduction of speaking to other people was accomplished in a progressive fashion. The child was first involved in talking to other individuals in a one-to-one setting. More people were gradually introduced until she was talking to small groups of adults and/or students. This generalization of speech was transferred to her classroom, and by the end of treatment she was speaking in her class before all the other students.

POSTTREATMENT

At the conclusion of her kindergarten year, the child was talking in school in a manner consistent with her peers. The child's parents and teacher completed posttreatment behavioral rating scales of her behaviors six months after she was initially evaluated. Where the rates had initially identified immaturity and withdrawal as areas of concern with her behavior, no rated behaviors existed at problematic levels on posttreatment evaluation. On the Burks' Behavior Rating Scale, none of the child's behaviors existed outside the not-significant range of functioning. On the Walker Problem Behavior Identification Checklist, none of her behaviors were rated above a t score of 57, with 60 being the cutoff for problematic functioning.

A six-month follow-up was conducted after the child had entered first grade. According to the child's teacher, she was talking openly in class in a manner consistent with her peers and had not manifested any behavioral concerns. The parents also reported that the child was talking in a manner consistent with her peers, and did not report the presence of any observable behavioral difficulties.

DISCUSSION

A 6-year-old girl who entered kindergarten and did not speak prompted this study. The disorder affecting her functioning had been identified as rare and disabling (APA 1994, Golwyn and Weinstock 1990), and it was. As she was not participating fully in classroom activities, her selective mutism hindered her school achievement and had strained her family relations.

The combination of extending Wilkens's (1985) distinction between transient and persistent selective mutism into an identification and treatment model, Porjes's (1992) learning theories treatment model, and the application of a multimodal treatment plan formed the basis for this project. Of primary importance in working with children displaying selective mutism is determining whether the disorder is a transient or persistent condition. Although the early identification of any disorder contributes to resolving difficulties as rapidly as possible (Nash et al. 1979), identifying and treating selective mutism represent two separate stages of treatment programming.

If the presented behavior is transient, monitoring is recommended because developmental maturation will likely resolve the selective mutism without interventions. When persistent selective mutism is presented, further evaluations are in order prior to interventions. If the evaluations indicate that the disorder is psychological in nature, then the application of Porjes's (1992) learning theory treatment model can be efficacious, as it was in this study.

The child displayed persistent selective mutism and a treatment plan was designed incorporating the child's parents, family, and teacher. The goal of the treatment was to increase her verbalizations. To this end, several behavioral techniques including shaping, positive reinforcement, desensitization, and modeling were utilized in conjunction with play therapy and family involvement in providing her treatment.

Following treatment the child spoke in a manner consistent with her peers. The other behavioral concerns that her parents and teacher had identified, immaturity and withdrawal, dissipated. A six-month follow-up, completed after the child had entered first grade, indicated that she was exhibiting speaking behaviors consistent with her peers without the presence of behavioral concerns.

Cunningham and colleagues (1983) indicated that there is a need for future research to determine the outcomes of various therapeutic combinations in the treatment of selective mutism. We hope that this study provides some insight into the troubling issue of what is effective in treating children with this disorder. Further investigation in distinguishing transient selective mutism from persistent selective mutism would also assist psychologists who are responsible for identifying and treating this puzzling disorder.

REFERENCES

Afnan, S., and Carr, A. (1989). Interdisciplinary treatment of a case of elective mutism. *British Journal of Occupational Therapy* 52:61–66.

Albert-Stewart, P. L. (1986). Positive reinforcement in short term treatment of an elective mute child: a case study. *Psychological Reports* 58:571–576.

American Psychiatric Association. (1994). *Diagnostic and Statistical Manual of Mental Disorders, Fourth Edition (DSM-IV)*. Washington, DC: American Psychiatric Association.

Atlas, J. A. (1993). Symbol use in a case of elective mutism. *Perceptual and Motor Skills* 76:1079–1082.

Atoynatan, T. H. (1986). Elective mutism: involvement of the mother in the treatment of the child. *Child Psychiatry and Human Development* 17:15–27.

Axline, V. M. (1947). *Play Therapy*. New York: Ballantine.

Barlow, K., Strother, J., and Landreth, G. (1986). Sibling group play therapy: an effective alternative with an electively mute child. *School Counselor* 34:44–50.

Black, B., and Uhde, T. W. (1992). Elective mutism as a variant of social phobia. *Journal of the American Academy of Child and Adolescent Psychiatry* 31:1090–1094.

Bozigar, J. A., and Hansen, R. A. (1984). Group treatment for electively mute children. *Social Work* 29:478–480.

Brown, B. J., and Lloyd, M. (1975). A controlled study of children not speaking at school. *Journal of the Association of Workers for Maladjusted Children* 3:49–63.

Cliffe, M. J. (1991). Behavioral modification by successive approximation: Saxon age example from Bede. *British Journal of Clinical Psychology* 30:367–369.

Cunningham, C. E., Cataldo, M. F., Mallion, C., and Keyes, J. B. (1983). A review and controlled single case evaluation of behavioral approaches to the management of elective mutism. *Child and Family Behavior Therapy* 5:25–49.

Friedman, R., and Karagan, N. (1973). Characteristics and management of elective mutism in children. *Psychology in the Schools* 10:249–252.

Golwyn, D. H., and Weinstock, R. C. (1990). Phenelzine treatment of elective mutism: a case report. *Journal of Clinical Psychiatry* 51:384–385.

Griffith, E. E., Schnelle, J. F., McNees, M. P., et al. (1975). Elective mutism in a first grader: the remediation of a complex behavioral problem. *Journal of Abnormal Child Psychology* 3:127–134.

Kehle, T. J., Owen, S. V., and Cressy, E. T. (1990). The use of self-modeling of an intervention in school psychology: a case study of elective mutism. *School Psychology Review* 19:115–121.

Klin, A., and Volkmar, F. R. (1993). Elective mutism and mental retardation. *Journal of the American Academy of Child and Adolescent Psychiatry* 32:860–864.

Kratochwill, T. (1981). *Selective Mutism: Implications for Research and Treatment*. Hillsdale, NJ: Erlbaum.

Kratochwill, T., Bordy, G., and Piersel, W. (1979). Elective mutism in children. In *Advances in Clinical Child Psychology*, vol. 2, ed. B. Lahey and A. Kazdin, pp. 194–240. New York: Plenum.

Krohn, D. D., Weckstein, S. M., and Wright, H. L. (1992). A study of the effectiveness of a specific treatment for elective mutism. *Journal of the American Academy of Child and Adolescent Psychiatry* 31:711–718.

Lumb, D., and Wolff, D. (1988). Mary doesn't talk. *British Journal of Special Education* 15:103–106.

Matson, J. L., Box, M. L., and Francis, K. L. (1992). Treatment of elective mute behavior in two developmentally delayed children using modeling and contingency management. *Journal of Behavior Therapy and Experimental Psychiatry* 23:221–229.

Nash, R. T., Thorpe, H. W., Andrews, M. M., and Davis, K. (1979). A management program for elective mutism. *Psychology in the Schools* 26:246–253.

Paniagua, F. A., and Saeed, M. A. (1988). A procedural distinction between elective and progressive mutism. *Journal of Behavior Therapy and Experimental Psychiatry* 19:207–210.

Porjes, M. D. (1992). Intervention with the selectively mute child. *Psychology in the Schools* 29:367–376.

Reed, J. B., and Mees, J. L. (1967). A marathon behavior modification programme of an electively mute child. *Journal of Child Psychology and Psychiatry* 8:27–30.

Rutter, M. (1977). Delayed speech. In *Child Psychiatry: Modern Approaches,* ed. M. Rutter and L. Hersov, pp. 698–716. Oxford: Blackwell Scientific.

Shreeve, D. F. (1991). Elective mutism: origins in stranger anxiety and selective attention. *Bulletin of the Menninger Clinic* 55:491–504.

Silver, L. B. (1985). Speech disorders. In *Comprehensive Textbook of Psychiatry,* ed. H. Kaplan and B. Sadock, 4th ed., pp. 1719–1721. Baltimore: Williams & Wilkens.

Tancer, N. K. (1992). Elective mutism: a review of the literature. In *Advances in Child Clinical Psychology,* vol. 14, ed. B. Lahey and D. Kazdin, pp. 265–288. New York: Plenum.

Watson, T. S., and Kramer, J. J. (1992). Multimethod behavioral treatment of long-term selective mutism. *Psychology in the Schools* 29:359–366.

Wilkens, R. (1985). A comparison of elective mutism and emotional disorders in children. *British Journal of Psychiatry* 146:198–203.

Wright, H. H., Miller, M. D., Cook, M. A., and Littman, J. R. (1985). Early identification and intervention with children who refuse to speak. *Journal of the American Academy of Child and Adolescent Psychiatry* 24:739–746.

Wright, H. W., Holmes, G. R., Cuccaro, M. L., and Leonhardt, T. V. (1994). A guided bibliography of the selective mutism (elective mutism) literature. *Psychological Reports* 74:995–1007.

PART II

BEHAVIOR THERAPY

4

INTERVENTION WITH THE SELECTIVELY MUTE CHILD

Michelle D. Porjes

REFERENCES TO CASES that involve children who selectively speak to a few individuals in specific environments dates back as far as 1877 when the terms *voluntary mutism* and *aphasia voluntaria* were used to describe children who were capable of speaking but were of their own will silent (Atoynatan 1986). In the 1930s, Kanner and Tramer coined the term *electiver mutismus* to define the behavior of children who were silent among everyone except for a small group of intimate relatives and peers (Louden 1987, Wilkens 1985). It was not until the 1950s, however, that the condition of being electively mute began to attract more attention from researchers and clinicians (Kolvin and Fundudis 1981).

Definitions of elective mutism include a number of criteria that distinguish the electively mute child from children exhibiting similar behaviors. According to *DSM-III-R* (American Psychiatric Association 1987), the diagnosis of elective mutism is determined by the presence of the following criteria: (1) the child continues to refuse to speak in one or more social situations, including school; (2) the child has the ability to speak and comprehend spoken language; and (3) the absence of speech is not due to another mental or physical disorder.

Silverman and Powers (1970) defined elective mutism in a similar manner to the *DSM-III-R* criteria. However, they also included in their definition additional criteria to distinguish elective mutism from other behaviors: (1) the child has exhibited the nonspeaking behavior for at least two years; (2) the child is of average intelligence; and (3) the child has been unresponsive to usual treatments. Though these definitions are somewhat vague in terms of specific criteria, they represent the foundation for determining the presence of elective mutism.

Regardless of the particular description, the underlying concept in these two definitions, as well as others, is that the "child does not speak in certain situations and/or to certain people" (Kratochwill 1981, p. 4). Louden (1987) reported that a common feature of electively mute children is that the children usually speak freely in selected environments.

Two types of elective mutism, transient and persistent, have been reported to exist (Wilkens 1985), although case studies of persistent elective mutism comprise a majority of the literature. This is primarily the case because the existence of electively mute children beyond the first two years of formal schooling is rather low (Kolvin and Fundudis 1981). In one survey of kindergarten children, 42 out of 6,072 children were reported to be not speaking in school eight weeks after school had started (Brown and Lloyd 1975). In a separate study done by Fundudis and colleagues (1979), 2 out of 3,300 children were reported to be electively mute at the age of 7 years. Because of the transient nature of selective mutism reported in these reviews, differences in terms of a gender ratio have been difficult to determine (Kolvin and Fundudis 1981). However, it is reported in *DSM-III-R* that the prevalence of selective mutism is slightly more common in girls than boys (American Psychiatric Association 1987).

Selectively mute children have been reported in several case studies to manifest a number of accompanying behaviors, including profound shyness (Wilkens 1985), little eye contact (Louden 1987), and enuresis (Barlow et al. 1986). Rutter (1977) referred to children who were selectively mute as withdrawn, timid, anxious, and even apathetic. It has also been suggested in several studies that behavioral problems such as oppositional behavior are common (Cunningham et al. 1983; Lesser-Katz 1988), and nonspeaking behavior has been known to be a precursor of more severe accompanying behavior problems (Kanner 1957). Kolvin and Fundudis (1981) reported that 71% of the electively mute children in their study displayed motor activity difficulties and bowel and bladder problems.

REVIEW OF THE LITERATURE

The literature on selective mutism has primarily fallen into two categories, case studies and reports, both of which deal with the effectiveness of treatment with selectively mute children (Friedman and Karagan 1973). However, regardless of the category, the specifics of selective mutism are described according to the theoretical orientation of the clinician. It is this theoretical orientation that sets the tone for the discussion on the major issues associated with selective mutism. Two general theoretical approaches, the psychoanalytic and the learning theory approach, exist in the literature. The approaches differ with respect to the etiology and the treatment of selective mutism.

PSYCHOANALYTIC APPROACHES

Several analytic theorists propose that the behavior of selective mutism is a manifestation of disturbed psychological processes. It has been suggested that selectively mute behavior is associated with neurotic reactions (Spieler 1944, in Wilkens 1985), psychological trauma occurring during one of the critical periods of language development (Cunningham et al. 1983), and a psychological fixation with nonspeaking behavior (Colligan et al. 1977).

It has also been suggested that selectively mute behavior originates as a function of family pathology (Atoynatan 1986, Bakwin and Bakwin 1972, Cunningham et al. 1983). Von Misch (1952, in Wilkens 1985) and others (Colligan et al. 1977; Parker et al. 1960) have suggested that the relationship between the mother and the selectively mute child is one in which the mother is overprotective and domineering and the child is overdependent and withdrawn. Atoynatan (1986) remarked that for selectively mute children, the mother–child relationship is one in which the child expresses the mother's hostility because the mother is overly timid. In return, the child gains an exclusive relationship with the mother. Elson and colleagues (1965) stipulated that the origin of selectively mute behavior lies in the combination of maternal rejection and paternal discomfort. These findings cited in the psychoanalytic literature are largely descriptive in nature, with the case study being the format of choice. The focus of the research is on the illustration and explanation of the underlying processes that cause the mute behavior.

In other psychoanalytic approaches the behavior of electing not to speak is viewed in terms of a return to instinctual survival techniques and lower order functioning. Selectively mute behavior is viewed in terms of a fixation with the anal stage of development in which not speaking is related to difficulties with this stage (Pustrom and Speers 1964, Redford 1977). Browne and colleagues (1963) saw selectively mute behavior as one of three parts of the "anal sulker" syndrome. The other two parts included the voluntary retention of urine and feces. The foundation for these various hypotheses comes from limited engagements with selectively mute children. No empirical support is reported in these studies for either the cause of the mutism or the following treatments that were employed: individual psychoanalytically based therapy (Redford 1977), family therapy (Pustrom et al. 1964), and joint mother-child therapy (Atoynatan 1986).

Among the studies described two factors are common: (1) selectively mute behavior is seen as a pathology rather than just one of the many behaviors exhibited by a child; and (2) the diagnosis of having the pathology "selective mutism" is assumed to reside strictly within the child. No credence is given to alternative explanations.

One final example of these factors comes from a clinician's notes of a 10-year-old selectively mute girl. The clinician hypothesized that the girl had stopped speaking when her father died "in order to freeze time, thereby denying his death and her own isolation" (Ambrosino 1979, in Atoynatan 1986).

LEARNING THEORY APPROACHES

An alternative approach to the etiology of selective mutism is found in the examination of the interaction between the selectively mute child and the child's environment. Learning theorists see nonverbal behavior as a learned response in which the refusal to speak is a method of manipulating the environment (Friedman and Karagan 1973). Reed and Mees (1967) were the first authors credited with the notion that selective mutism may be the result of a learned pattern of behavior. They suggested that the nonverbal behavior was being maintained by social reinforcement from significant others in the child's environment, such as parents and teachers. Thus, in order to break the cycle of nonverbal behavior, the social environment needed to be "reprogrammed."

Reed and Mees (1967) used a combination of systematic desensitization and fading-in techniques with a 6-year-old selectively mute girl. They hypothesized that in the presence of strangers, nonverbal behavior would occur. Consequently, they established a contingency system whereby the girl was required to speak to her mother in order to receive something she desired. With the gradual introduction of strangers into the girl's environment while she was speaking, speech in the presence of strangers was established. The results indicated that in a relatively short period of time the rate of speech increased and was generalized to new situations.

Given this alternative view of the etiology of selective mutism, the interventions employed in past case studies have reflected the belief that a change in the environment's response to a child's nonverbal behavior will significantly increase verbal behavior and its overall generalization. Operant conditioning procedures such as reinforcement in the form of contingency management, shaping and stimulus fading (Albert-Stewart 1986, Bednar 1974, Colligan et al. 1977, Lipton 1980, Louden 1987, Rosenbaum and Kellman 1973), escape-avoidance techniques, and aversive contingencies (Cunningham et al. 1983) have all been reported in the literature.

Many studies report the use of two or more of these techniques together to enhance the production of speech (Colligan et al. 1977, Rosenbaum and Kellman 1973). In one study, stimulus fading and contingency management techniques were used with a 6-year-old selectively mute girl. The girl was required to whisper a response to a question in order to receive a bead that would be used to make a necklace. As success with the shaping techniques increased, the volume at which the girl was required to respond also increased until the girl was communicating at an acceptable volume and rate (Lipton 1980). Bednar (1974) also employed similar techniques of shaping and contingency management in the intervention with a 10-year-old selectively mute boy in which he earned coins as a form of reinforcement. By dividing speech into a series of successive steps, conversation was approximated at a rate in which success was frequently experienced by the selectively mute child.

What makes the term *selective mutism* (as opposed to *elective mutism*) more appropriate to this phenomenon is the selective nature of the behavior. Not only does the child elect when to speak, but the child selects the conditions under which to speak. Under those conditions in which the child is given the choice to speak or remain nonverbal, selectively mute children chose when to speak, where to speak, and to whom to speak. Because of this "selective" verbal behavior, the term *selective mutism*, which more distinctly describes this type of behavior, will be used for the duration of this paper.

CASE STUDIES

This section discusses the interventions used with two selectively mute children. Although the interventions used with each child varied slightly, the underlying principles upon which the interventions were based are the same. These case studies used the learning theory perspective, which suggests that selective mutism is a learned behavior that has been reinforced over time.

The two cases presented here are not designed to provide the step-by-step procedure that was undertaken with each child. Rather, the cases are presented to provide the reader with an overview of several guidelines used in the interventions. Consistent with the learning theory approach, these guidelines included the analysis of those factors that maintained the nonverbal behavior, the reformation of the environment's response to the nonverbal behavior, the successive approximation of speech in stages, and the generalization of speech to new conditions. These guidelines also provide the theoretical foundation upon which the four stages of the intervention plan were established: (1) an ecological analysis, (2) compilation of the reinforcement menus, (3) elicitation of initial speech, and (4) generalization of speech to new situations and new people.

In both instances, the author designed the intervention plan and collected the data. The intervention plan was implemented by the author together with the teacher and other significant people in each child's environment.

SUBJECTS

Subject one (S-1) and subject two (S-2) were both 6-year-olds in the first grade. They were enrolled in separate public schools in Colorado.

S-1, a female, was the younger of two children in the family. S-1 was reported by the mother to have exhibited selectively mute behavior since her preschool years. The mother had attempted to set some requirements for speech during S-1's preschool years, but the child's pediatrician advised against setting limits for speech. Following the advice from the pediatrician, the mother stopped setting the requirements for speech. At home, the mother reported that the child would not comply with her requests. In addition, S-1 engaged in frequent tantrum episodes, which included hitting, kicking, and biting.

S-1 was seen by a psychiatrist for a 1-year period to uncover reasons behind her nonverbal behavior and to engage the child in speech. During this time no speech occurred. Several short-term interventions were tried with S-1 in kindergarten by the school's speech therapist. This resulted in some speech outside the classroom setting with three to four other children present, but the speech that resulted from these interventions did not transfer to the classroom situation.

S-1 was placed in a regular first-grade classroom with special services in the form of speech therapy provided. According to the teacher, her academic performance was acceptable. S-1 would complete writing and arithmetic assignments, but she would not read aloud or answer teacher-directed questions aloud. The only verbal behavior that occurred during the school day was when S-1 would whisper directly into the ear of her teacher or a female classmate.

Outside of the school and home settings, S-1 was inconsistent with verbal speech. She would sometimes speak face to face with a peer at the other child's home. Occasionally, S-1 would order aloud her food at a restaurant. However, she would not speak in the presence of large groups of children. During her Brownie troop meetings, for instance, S-1 did not engage in any face-to-face verbal behavior.

S-2, a male, was a younger child of several children. S-2 was placed in a self-contained individualized program (SCIP) in which he was also integrated into a regular first-grade classroom during the school day for subjects such as art, computers, and social studies. He had been transferred to his present school about 2 months after the school year had begun. At the commencement of the intervention, S-2 had been in the present school for about 2½ months.

S-2 was reported by the previous school psychologist, in a series of case notes, to have been selectively mute since he had begun kindergarten. He was subjected to frequent mild ear infections and a slight hearing loss was possible. No interventions were reported by previous school personnel to have been tried.

The SCIP teacher reported that S-2 would complete assignments and tasks with consistently correct results. Both the SCIP classroom teacher and the regular first-grade teacher reported that S-2 would comply with all requests except for requests for speech. No verbalizations, other than laughing aloud, were reported. The SCIP teacher had been able to convince S-2 to touch his tongue to the roof of his mouth in order to receive a lunch ticket.

PROCEDURE

As suggested above, the procedures used in both cases were broken down into four stages. Each stage represented an important step in the intervention sequence.

Stage 1: An ecological analysis. In an attempt to operationalize the principles of learning theory, an ecological analysis of each situation was undertaken. The ecological analysis used in these cases is similar to the behavioral antecedent-behavior-consequences method. In the ecological analysis, the cues found in the environment that help maintain the behavior are examined, including any responses to the child's nonverbal behavior by the environment. Not only are the consequences analyzed, but also the reaction of the individual to the consequences. For example, the feedback (either positive or negative) given to the nonverbal behavior is examined together with the child's response to this feedback.

At the outset, the selectively mute behavior was not seen as an indication of pathology. Instead, the nonverbal behavior was interpreted to be adaptive and functional. In some way, the nonverbal behavior served a purpose for each child (Macht 1990). The exact purpose that the selectively mute behavior served is extremely difficult to pinpoint. Yet, both children were able to acquire what they needed in school with use of gestures to classmates and teachers.

Because the nonverbal behavior was not viewed as pathological, the focus of the intervention was not on the cause of the selectively mute behavior, but rather on the factors that maintained the nonverbal behavior. The intervention involved determining the conditions under which the nonverbal behavior was most and least likely to occur. These conditions were determined through the ecological analysis that was executed in both cases. This analysis involved examining those factors in the interaction between each child and his or her environment that were maintaining the nonverbal behavior.

In both cases, the feedback given to each child for the nonverbal behavior by teachers/classmates was neutral or perhaps viewed as positive by the child. This was demonstrated by the child's reaction to the feedback and his or her choice to remain nonverbal. Both classroom teachers observed that when a question was asked of the selectively mute child, other classmates would intercept the question and remark that the child was "shy" or "didn't like to talk." Without an understanding of the processes that occur in the interactions between the child and his or her environment, the choice of interventions would have been guesses at best.

Once the factors that were maintaining the behavior were determined, the actual intervention plan was devised. In order to increase the desired verbal behavior, changes in the system were made. The ecological analysis conducted on each child provided the information about what changes should be implemented and where they should occur. The adults involved provided the children with positive feedback when the children engaged in verbal behavior. Then a contingency system that tied speech or approximations to speech to desired activities was established. When the children did not engage in verbal behavior, those involved provided the children with negative feedback in terms of withdrawing what was valued or desired by the children. In both cases, until intervention was undertaken, there seemed to be no reason for either child to become verbal. Only when changes in the feedback part of the system were implemented did verbalizations start to occur.

Stage 2: Compilation of the reinforcement menus. For both children, a list of reinforcers was compiled before the intervention process began. Gathering powerful reinforcers was an important part of the process because reinforcers are only useful if they are of value to the child (Bednar 1974). The reinforcement list, also known as a reinforcement menu, included those activities/things that each child enjoyed. The items listed on the reinforcement menus were strongly linked to the issue of compliance with speech. In these two cases, gaining what was valued was contingent upon the production of speech or approximations thereof. By not engaging in the verbal behavior, the child presumably lost access to what was valued.

For S-1, the teacher and the mother each compiled a list that included both home and school activities that S-1 had been reported to enjoy. S-1's list consisted of activities such as recess, coloring, riding her bike, watching videos, and playing with friends. Previous to the intervention, these activities were "free" and available to the child on a continual basis.

In the case of S-2, the SCIP teacher and the child's regular teacher each compiled lists. Tangible reinforcers were used with S-2. The list included items such as candy, stickers, balloons, and games. The reinforcers were used as a method to increase the amount of verbalizations. Eventually, the list was broadened to include classroom reinforcers (e.g., computers, free time).

Stage 3: Elicitation of initial speech. Interventions utilizing a combination of a contingency management system and shaping procedures have generally been successful in the increase and maintenance of verbal behavior (Albert-Stewart 1986, Bednar 1974, Colligan et al. 1977, Rosenbaum and Kellman 1973). Given the success of these past interventions, a similar system was employed with each child in this study.

A contingency management system was used to convey to each child that "when you do the behavior requested of you, you gain what you desire" and "when you do not do the behavior requested of you, you do not gain what you desire." In some respects, the previous contingencies set by others for the children were backwards. That is, the message of "when you do not talk, you still get what you want" was communicated to the children by the environment. Under a new system, the children were required to engage in verbal behavior in order to attain what was valued. In this new system, expectations for verbal behavior were communicated by the adults in each child's environment.

Although shaping procedures have been used in several case studies involving selectively mute children to approximate speech, little mention is made of the starting point for the shaping. In both of the present cases, shaping began at a point where each child had the necessary skills to comply with the request. The level at which a child can succeed at the task near or at 100% of the time is known as the child's present performance level (PPL; Macht 1975). By determining the child's PPL, the question of ability is ruled out as a possibility and compliance remains the central issue. Also, commencing shaping procedures at the child's PPL increases the probability of success.

The rate at which subsequent shaping procedures were introduced and the decision to move ahead in the shaping process also was related to the issue of PPL because the PPL changed as the intervention process continued. At each stage in the shaping process, a new PPL was established. The decision to continue the shaping process at the next level was made when the current shaping technique was occurring consistently.

S-1 was required to engage in some sort of verbal behavior (e.g., make a sound, say a word, talk to a teacher or another child) in order to participate or gain what she enjoyed at school and at home. Consequently, when she did not engage in the verbal behavior she did not gain what she valued.

The shaping procedure used with S-1 involved approximating vocal speech with an initial step and several intermediary steps. The mother reported that S-1 would engage in conversation on the phone on a regular basis. A previous baseline taken by the author demonstrated that S-1 would talk to the author on the phone in other situations. Her PPL involved speech on the phone outside of the school building. A phone shaping procedure was undertaken in the school as the initial step of the procedure. The process involved talking on the phone after school hours with various individuals (author, secretaries, teachers, etc.) and then talking on the phone in the presence of others.

The intervention with S-2 was conducted in a one-on-one situation and it also involved shaping procedures used in conjunction with simple contingencies. S-2's initial PPL was engaging in oral gestures, such as sticking out his tongue. Therefore, the initial phase of intervention involved these oral gestures. Once these oral gestures were occurring consistently, S-2 was then required to whisper sounds ("puh," "wa"), whisper words ("hi," "yea"), and eventually use vocal speech. The contingencies used with S-2 were tied into the activity that was underway (e.g., "Say 'yea,' then you can continue coloring on the board").

Stage 4: Generalization of speech to new situations and new people. One of the most difficult stages in the intervention with selectively mute children is the generalization of speech to new situations and new environments. In both cases, the generalization of speech became important after speech upon request was occurring frequently.

Once S-1 was consistently talking on the phone, the generalization phase of the intervention was implemented. This phase involved eliciting speech from S-1 in the presence of teachers and other students in various parts of the school building. This procedure was first conducted after the regular school day in the school building and then replicated during the school hours.

Once speech for S-2 was consistent in a one-on-one situation, the focus of the intervention turned to replicating speech with others by introducing individuals such as teachers and classmates into the one-on-one situation. The final step in the generalization process for S-2 involved replicating speech, also by utilizing shaping procedures, into both of S-2's class environments.

Everyone who came in contact with either child during the school day was involved in the intervention process. Teachers and other school personnel (secretaries, music teacher, physical education teacher) set contingencies for speech for each child in which a verbal response was required. In both cases, the primary teachers were responsible for monitoring the compliance with these contingencies.

For both subjects, the intervention involved short sessions that were provided on a frequent and predictable basis. Feedback was also provided frequently to the children and all of the individuals involved in both interventions. In addition, provisions were made for dealing with a return to nonverbal behavior or a "shut down." A "shut down" was defined as the cessation of speech during the intervention time or after the intervention was completed. The provisions involved the loss of valued activities when the subjects returned to nonverbal behavior.

RESULTS

Currently, S-1 continues to speak in a quiet voice in the classroom setting on a consistent basis. She speaks face to face to the other children in the class and she will answer the teacher's questions aloud when requested to do so. She volunteers to answer questions in group discussions and reads aloud for the teacher. S-1 has access to all of the activities on her reinforcement menu as long as she speaks in a voice at school. Consequences, in the form of a loss of activities, still exist for a return to nonverbal behavior.

S-2 uses speech with teachers in both classrooms, although speech is often in response to requests made by the teachers. In the SCIP classroom, S-2 reads aloud in front of small groups of children. He will also engage in speech with other school personnel. One of the school secretaries reported that S-2 had come into the office and asked her where his class was when he could not find them. A contingency remains in effect for S-2 in which he must respond to a teacher's question or request for speech and acknowledge his teachers with a verbal response when he sees them in other parts of the school building. Losing activities that he values is the consequence for not complying. When S-2 engages in verbal behavior at school, he continues to have access to the activities he values.

DISCUSSION

From a research orientation, an important limitation of this chapter is the descriptive nature of the case studies. The integrity of the interventions used would have been increased if data in terms of verbal behavior were provided. Rather than charting the increases in verbal behavior and the conditions under which the verbal behavior occurred, the specifics of the interventions came from the author's case notes. Future research on selective mutism should strive to be more experimental in nature by documenting the changes in verbal behavior over time and the conditions under which they occurred. An additional limitation of this study is the failure to have follow-up data. Due to uncontrollable circumstances, the long-term effects of the interventions in maintaining speech are unknown.

With these limitations in mind, however, the approach outlined here does provide a practical framework for the school psychologist and others who work in the school setting to use when faced with a selectively mute child. Although the precise procedure used with each child will vary, the rationale and sequence of the intervention process will remain the same. It is the method outlined in the two case studies that will aid the school psychologist and others in planning the intervention process and coordinating the school personnel. The success of increasing verbal behavior in the school setting with the selectively mute child depends on a systematic, coordinated approach.

It is important to begin the intervention process as soon as a selectively mute child is identified for two reasons. First, the chances of success are greater when the child is younger and in an earlier grade. The amount of time the child has been nonverbal is less than that of an older child who has remained nonverbal in school for a greater amount of time. It becomes increasingly harder to change the nonverbal behavior because of the increased amount of time the child has spent in school and the presumed social reinforcement for the nonverbal behavior.

The second reason is related to the time of intervention and is also of great concern for school psychologists. This is the relationship between the selectively mute behavior and learning at school. In these two cases, as in many other cases involving selectively mute children, the nonverbal behavior hampered academic assessment. Because of the lack of verbal feedback on the part of each child, both teachers reported some questions as to where each child was in regard to reading and language arts. Without knowledge of where a child is functioning academically, it becomes difficult to know if remediation is needed and where it should occur. As a child remains selectively mute, academic difficulties can go undetected and turn into more severe academic problems in the future, even if the child is then speaking in the school setting.

ACKNOWLEDGMENTS

The author gratefully acknowledges Dr. Joel Macht for his support and guidance with these two cases and Dr. Howard Knoff for his helpful comments during the preparation of this paper.

REFERENCES

Albert-Stewart, P. L. (1986). Positive reinforcement in short-term treatment of an electively mute child: a case study. *Psychological Reports* 58:571–576.

American Psychiatric Association (1987). *Diagnostic and Statistical Manual of Mental Disorders, Third Edition, Revised (DSM-III-R)*. Washington, DC: American Psychiatric Association.

Atoynatan, T. H. (1986). Elective mutism: involvement of the mother in the treatment of the child. *Child Psychiatry and Human Development* 17(1):15–27.

Bakwin, H., and Bakwin, R. M. (1972). *Behavior Disorders in Children*. Philadelphia: W. B. Saunders.

Barlow, K., Strother, J., and Landreth, G. (1986). Sibling group play therapy: an alternative with the electively mute child. *School Counselor* 34(1):44–50.

Bednar, R. A. (1974). A behavioral approach to treating an elective mute in the school. *Journal of School Psychology* 12(4):326–337.

Brown, B. J., and Lloyd, M. (1975). A controlled study of children not speaking at school. *Journal of the Association of Workers for Maladjusted Children* 3:49–63.

Browne, E., Wilson, V., and Laybourne, P. (1963). Diagnosis and treatment of elective mutism in children. *Journal of the American Academy of Child Psychiatry* 2:605–617.

Colligan, R. W., Colligan, R. C., and Dillard, M. K. (1977). Contingency management in the classroom treatment of long-term elective mutism: a case report. *Journal of School Psychology* 15(1):9–17.

Cunningham, C. E., Cataldo, M. F., Mallion, C., and Keyes, J. B. (1983). A review and controlled single case evaluation of behavioral approaches to the management of elective mutism. *Child and Family Behavior Therapy* 5(4):25–49.

Elson, A., Pearson, C., Jones, C. D., and Schumacher, E. (1965). Follow-up study of childhood elective mutism. *Archives of General Psychiatry* 13:182–187.

Friedman, R., and Karagan, N. (1973). Characteristics and management of elective mutism in children. *Psychology in the Schools* 10(2):249–252.

Fundudis, T., Kolvin, I., and Gardise, R. F. (1979). *Speech Retarded and Deaf Children: Their Psychological Development*. London: Academic Press.

Kanner, L. (1957). *Child Psychiatry*, 3rd ed. Springfield, IL: Charles C Thomas.

Kolvin, I., and Fundudis, T. (1981). Elective mute children: Psychological development and background factors. *Journal of Child Psychology and Psychiatry* 22(3):219–232.

Kratochwill, T. (1981). *Selective Mutism: Implications for Research and Treatment*. Hillsdale, NJ: Lawrence Erlbaum.

Lesser-Katz, M. (1988). The treatment of elective mutism as stranger reaction. *Psychotherapy* 25(2):305–313.

Lipton, H. (1980). Rapid reinstatement of speech using stimulus fading with a selectively mute child. *Journal of Behavioral Therapy and Experimental Psychiatry* 11:147–149.

Louden, D. M. (1987). Elective mutism: a case study of a disorder of childhood. *Journal of the Medical Association* 79(10):1043–1048.

Macht, J. E. (1975). *Teacher/Teachim: The Toughest Game in Town*. New York: Wiley.

———— (1990). *Managing Classroom Behavior: An Ecological Approach to Academic and Social Learning*. New York: Longman.

Parker, E. B., Olsen, T., and Throckmorton, M. (1960). Social casework with elementary schoolchildren who do not talk in school. *Social Work* 5:64–70.

Pustrom, E., and Speers, R. W. (1964). Elective mutism in children. *Journal of the American Academy of Child Psychiatry* 3:287–297.

Redford, P. A. (1977). Psychoanalytically based therapy as the treatment of choice for a six-year-old elective mute. *Journal of Child Psychotherapy* 4:49–65.

Reed, J. B., and Mees, J. L. (1967). A marathon behavior modification programme of an elective mute child. *Journal of Child Psychology and Psychiatry* 8:27–30.

Rosenbaum, E., and Kellman, M. (1973). Treatment of a selectively mute third-grade child. *Journal of School Psychology* 11(1):26–29.

Rutter, M. (1977). Delayed speech. In *Child Psychiatry: Modern Approaches*, ed. M. Rutter and L. Hersov, pp. 698–716. Oxford: Blackwell Scientific.

Silverman, G., and Powers, D. F. (1970). Elective mutism in children. *Medical College of Virginia Quarterly* 6:149–152.

Wilkens, R. (1985). A comparison of elective mutism and emotional disorders in children. *British Journal of Psychiatry* 146:198–203.

5

ELECTIVE MUTISM: SPECIAL TREATMENT OF A SPECIAL CASE

Anders Lysne

THE START BARRIER

The main barrier to overcome in a therapeutic setting for a child who suffers from true elective mutism is the first verbal responding. In addition to the intrapsychic resistance to start speaking, the child is reluctant to draw attention to him- or herself by giving up the role as the silent child. The initiation phase is always the most difficult, because reinforcement does not start to work before the first verbal responding has come. Hence, response-initiation procedures are a very important part of a behavioral-treatment program.

In a review of the literature about behavioral treatment of elective mutism, Labbe and Williamson (1984) refer to studies where the use of escape or avoidance procedure has been reported as being effective in producing initial verbalizations (Crema and Kerr 1978, Halpern et al. 1971, Piersel and Kratochwill 1981, Williamson et al. 1977).

Escape procedures put much pressure on the mute child, and they can be a painful experience. For this reason they should not be used at too early an age, and they should never be the first method used. If such a method fails, it might also reinforce the resistance to start speaking. Therefore, it is important to create a trustful relationship between the implementing person and the client before escape procedures are used. Generally speaking, such methods should not be recommended unless the child is judged to be mentally strong enough to take the pressure, and there should be a convincing probability of a positive outcome.

CASE CHARACTERISTICS

The case reported here is of a 14-year-old boy, raised in an ordinary family together with two older brothers who have not shown any speech problems. The mother is child centered and very overprotective toward her youngest boy. The father appeared detached from his family, and he finally left the home when the youngest boy was 10 years old. During the last two years the boy has had a "stepfather" in his mother's man-friend, who has lived in the house, and to whom he was able to start talking after some months.

The boy had several attacks of false croup when he was a baby, and he was hospitalized for two weeks when he was 1 year old. This was a traumatic event for the child. When awake, he constantly cried for his mother, and he showed, while in the hospital, severe signs of separation anxiety.

His speech and language development seemed normal until the age of 4, when he became reluctant to speak outside of his home. After some weeks, he only spoke to the family members at home, and he refused to talk when anybody else came to the house. He spoke three times at home when he was unaware that a visitor had dropped in. When he detected what had happened, he first became very sad, and after a while he acted with despair and aggression. Once he had spoken a few words by mistake to his male cousin, and after this he refused to see him for two years.

The boy has not appeared particularly uneasy or anxious, but his mother reported that he had always been reluctant to go to bed and to fall asleep at night—a kind of sleep phobia—because he was afraid of bad dreams and nightmares, from which he frequently suffered. After he started to speak, he confirmed in interview that the nightmares were a threat to him, and at times he was so afraid that he had to sleep with his mother.

At home he was active and devoted to his mother and brothers, but he could be angry and he was sometimes aggressive. He could play outside his home with some close friends in the neighborhood, but he was always silent. At school he was quiet and kind, compliant and cooperative in following class routines. He did not show the most commonly observed behavioral features associated with elective mutism such as shyness and manipulative strategies. The boy was well accepted by his classmates, and he was well adjusted to them. These classmates never challenged him to start talking. Keeping silent seemed to be easy and natural to him.

BASELINE AND ASSESSMENT

The boy met the two *DSM-III-R* diagnostic criteria for elective mutism (American Psychiatric Association 1987). He was totally silent outside his home, despite his ability to comprehend spoken language and to speak. Tape recordings of his speech at home showed that he had a normal voice with distinct articulation, and age-appropriate vocabulary. According to his mother's report, he had started to talk about the same age as his two older brothers, and his speech development seemed normal. Her worry started when she detected that the boy constantly refused to speak outside the home, but she did not inform the school or any other authority about her son's silence until some months before he started school at the age of 7.

During the first year at school, the boy was regularly seen by the school psychologist and a speech pathologist. At the end of the first year, a referral was made to the local psychiatric clinic for children and youth. For a couple of years the boy was seen by a therapist once a week in the school setting, and for one month he and his mother stayed at the institution. No improvement could be observed. The boy was then included in the author's research program, and a group of professionals under the author's leadership took responsibility for further treatment.

His scholastic aptitude was informally estimated to be above average; this was confirmed to some extent by a score close to the average on Raven's standard progressive matrices test. Because of his speech handicap, the boy received much extra support from an assistant class teacher.

TREATMENT

A contingency management program was implemented in the school setting by the class teacher, instructed and supervised by the project leader. As the boy was a true elective mutist, the main problem was to initiate his first verbal responding outside his home. He was strongly resistant to all interventions, and after a while a variety of behavioral treatment approaches were tried in order to initiate verbalization, such as stimulus fading, response cost and reinforcement sampling (Beech et al. 1993, Labbe and Williamson 1984, Piersel and Kratochwill 1981). The method designed by David Premack (Homme 1970) was thought to be worth trying, but none of these methods proved to have the power of releasing the first word.

When it seemed likely that the boy would continue as the "silent boy," at least throughout his school years, it was decided to try an escape procedure. Such a method is usually not recommended, because it might have serious short-term and/or long-term consequences. Treatment always includes some risks and ethical problems. In this case special precautions were taken, and an extensive assessment was made of how the boy was most likely to react to an escape procedure. He had been closely observed for years in different treatment situations, and the parents and all who were involved in his case agreed that an escape procedure would probably help him overcome the barriers and that it should not hurt him seriously.

Three interventions were planned and introduced as a training program to be held at his school, based on an agreement between the boy and the conductor. A response goal was defined for each setting. The goals for the two first settings were to imitate sounds made by known animals, sheep and dogs, which the boy had been able to accomplish a few times before. For the third setting, the goal was that the boy should emit one single word before termination of the session.

The boy was very reluctant to imitate the animal sounds after the conductor's voice in the first and second settings, but he was finally able to do so. The third session was most difficult both for the boy and the conductor. It took time before the boy really understood that he would not be released from the setting before he had emitted at least one word. He tried to press out some sounds, which were not accepted as words. Finally, to the question, "Do you want to go home?" he answered, "Yes." This word response was reinforced verbally and by the sharing of some chocolate with the conductor. This was the turning point. The next day he was willing to continue with the training program. The boy seemed happy with the breakthrough with his speech problem, and he made rapid progress during the following days. In a couple of weeks he was able to speak like everyone else at his school and in his social life. After ten years of silence outside his home, he achieved the ability to speak to any person in any situation at the age of 14.

DISCUSSION

The boy represents an interesting case of elective mutism. He met the two *DSM-III-R* diagnostic criteria as a true elective mutist, but he was atypical in his personality traits and in the associated features of behavior that are most commonly found in electively mute children (Black and Uhde 1992, Hartmann 1993, Krohn et al. 1992). He appeared open and kind, compliant and cooperative, and he was seldom shy, openly anxious, avoiding, suspicious, or manipulative.

In interviews held after he started to speak, he has been open about how he experienced his mutism. According to his description, it functioned on a conscious level, at least partly. He knew he would not speak to anybody when leaving home. Silence would come automatically, but he did watch out when provoked by someone to speak. He did not need to keep in mind every minute that he should be silent, and he was never afraid that he spontaneously would have a slip of the tongue.

Speedy elimination of true elective mutism which has lasted for years is rare. Only a few cases have been reported (Reid et al. 1967, Wergeland 1979). Behavior-modification therapy for elective mutism has to be extended, as a rule, over a fairly long period of time, and progress may be slow. In contrast, intervention at an early age, shortly after mutism has commenced, can be effective, as has been shown in a study by Wright et al. (1985). It is important, therefore, to start treatment as soon as possible after diagnosis. Later in life, some elective mutes may eventually outgrow their handicap (Wergeland 1979), but until such time they will be severely deprived of important stimulation in their intellectual and social growth.

SUMMARY

A 14-year-old boy, who had stopped using verbal language outside his home at the age of 4, was diagnosed as electively mute in connection with an epidemiological-longitudinal research program (Rutter 1982) conducted in Norway during 1989–92. The treatment program, based on principles for contingency management, was carried out in school by the class teacher, and instructed and supervised by the project leader, who also saw the boy and his mother regularly. The boy was compliant and cooperative in following the treatment procedures, but he was strongly resistant to behavioral interventions aimed at initiating verbal responding (Labbe and Williamson 1984). The treatment became a "game" where he was always the winner, with an adverse reinforcing effect (Sluckin et al. 1991). New approaches had to be tried, and finally an escape procedure (Piersel and Kratochwill 1981) released the first verbal responding outside his home. After a couple of weeks he had achieved normal speech at school and also in his social life.

REFERENCES

American Psychiatric Association. (1987). *Diagnostic and Statistical Manual of Mental Disorders, Third Edition Revised (DSM-III-R)*. Washington, DC: American Psychiatric Association.

Beech, J. R., Harding, L., and Hilton-Jones, D. (1993). *Assessments in Speech and Language Therapy*. New York: Routledge Assessment Library.

Black, B., and Uhde, T. (1992). Elective mutism as a variant of social phobia. *Journal of the Academy of Child and Adolescent Psychiatry* 31:1090-1094.

Crema, J. E., and Kerr, J. M. (1978). Elective mutism: a child care case study. *Child Care Quarterly* 1:215-226.

Halpern, W. J., Hammond, I., and Cohen, R. (1971). A therapeutic approach to speech phobia: elective mutism reexamined. *Journal of the Academy of Child Psychiatry* 10:94-107.

Hartmann, B. (1993). *Mutismus. Zur Theorie und Kasuistik des totalen und elektiven Mutismus. Schriften zur Sprachheilpädagogik*, Band 1, pp. 1-127. Berlin: Spiess.

Homme, L. (1970). *How to Use Contingency Contracting in the Classroom*. Champaign, IL: Research Press.

Kratochwill, T. R. (1981). *Selective Mutism: Implications for Research and Treatment*. Hillsdale, NJ: Erlbaum.

Krohn, D. D., Wechstein, S. M., and Wright, H. L. (1992). A study of the effectiveness of a specific treatment for elective mutism. *Journal of the Academy of Child and Adolescent Psychiatry* 31:711-718.

Labbe, E. E., and Williamson, D. A. (1984). Behavioral treatment of elective mutism: a review of the literature. *Clinical Psychology Review* 4:273-292.

Piersel, W. C., and Kratochwill, T. R. (1981). A teacher-implemented contingency management package to assess and treat selective mutism. *Behavioral Assessment* 3:371-382.

Reid, J. B., Hawkins, M., Keutzer, C., et al. (1967). A marathon behavior modification programme of an elective mute child. *Journal of Child Psychology and Psychiatry* 8:27-30.

Rutter, M. (1982). Epidemiological-longitudinal approaches to the study of development. In *The Concept of Development*, Minne-

sota Symposia on Child Psychology, vol. 15, ed. W. A. Collins, pp. 105–144. Hillsdale, NJ: Erlbaum.

Sluckin, A., Foreman, N., and Herbert, M. (1991). Behavioural treatment programs and selectivity of speaking at follow-up in sample of 25 selective mutes. *Australian Psychiatry* 26:132–137.

Wergeland, H. (1979). Elective mutism. *Acta Psychiatrica Scandinavica* 59:218–228.

Williamson, D. A., Sanders, S. H., Sewell, W. R., et al. (1977). The behavioral treatment of elective mutism: two case studies. *Journal of Behavior Therapy and Experimental Psychiatry* 8:143–149.

Wright, H. L., Miller, D., Cook, M. A., and Littman, J. (1985). Early identification and intervention with children who refuse to speak. *Journal of the Academy of Child and Adolescent Psychiatry* 24:739–746.

6

COMBINING SELF-MODELING AND STIMULUS FADING IN THE TREATMENT OF AN ELECTIVELY MUTE CHILD

Grayson N. Holmbeck and John V. Lavigne

THE ESSENTIAL FEATURE of elective mutism is the "persistent refusal to talk in one or more major social situations (including at school)" (*DSM-III-R*, American Psychiatric Association 1987, p. 89) in a child who has the ability to speak and comprehend spoken language. Although not included in the diagnostic criteria of the *DSM-III-R*, other personality and familial characteristics have also been identified: excessive shyness, anxiety, social isolation and withdrawal, maternal overprotection, a symbiotic relationship with a parent (usually the mother), language difficulties, early hospitalization or trauma, marital disharmony, fear of strangers, depression, and a manipulative, controlling, or aggressive interpersonal style (Hayden 1980, Kolvin and Fundudis 1981, Lesser-Katz 1986, 1988, Meyers 1984, Rutter and Garmezy 1983, Wilkins 1985, Wright et al. 1985).

Based on a review of 68 cases, Hayden (1980) identified four subtypes of elective mutism: symbiotic mutism (characterized by a symbiotic relationship with a caregiver and a manipulative and negativistic attitude toward controlling adults), speech phobic mutism (characterized by a fear of hearing one's voice accompanied by obsessive-compulsive behaviors), reactive mutism (caused by a single traumatic event or a series of traumatic events and characterized by depression and withdrawal), and passive-aggressive mutism (characterized by a defiant refusal to speak and the use of "silence as a weapon"). Similarly, Lesser-Katz (1988) discusses two types of elective mutism: a compliant, timid, anxious, dependent, and insecure subtype and a noncompliant, passive-aggressive, and avoidant subtype.

In addition to these diagnostic and typological discussions, there have been numerous reports of successful treatments for elective mutism. Treatment approaches vary widely with respect to theoretical perspective and the techniques employed (see Kratochwill et al. 1979, and Labbe and Williamson 1984, for reviews). These procedures include: (1) behavioral shaping and operant conditioning (e.g., Albert-Stewart 1986, Bednar 1974, Colligan et al. 1977, Morin et al. 1982, Nash et al. 1979, Nolan and Pence 1970, Sanok and Striefel 1979), (2) avoidance conditioning (van der Kooy and Webster 1975), (3) punishment (e.g., Wulbert et al. 1973), (4) self-modeling (Dowrick and Hood 1978, Kehle et al. 1990, Pigott and Gonzales 1987), (5) stimulus fading (e.g., Conrad et al. 1974, Lipton 1980, Reid et al. 1967, Richards and Hansen 1978, Rosenbaum and Kellman 1973, Williamson et al. 1977, Wulbert et al. 1973), (6) family interventions (Atoynatan 1986, Hoffman and Laub 1986, Lazarus et al. 1983, Meyers 1984, Rosenberg and Lindblad 1978), (7) individual psychotherapy (e.g., Wergeland 1979), (8) psychodynamic approaches (Chethik 1973, Lesser-Katz 1986, 1988), and (9) sibling group play therapy (Barlow et al. 1986).

Although effective, many of these treatment strategies are extremely time-consuming and costly (see Lipton 1980, and Reid et al. 1967, for exceptions). For example, Bednar's (1974) operant approach required fifteen months of treatment, Richards and Hansen's (1978) stimulus fading strategy required fifty-five treatment sessions and twenty-five consultation visits, and Wergeland (1979) reported that some children with elective mutism required four years of individual psychotherapy or even psychiatric hospitalization. In an attempt to shorten the duration and cost of treatment, some have attempted to combine two or more approaches to enhance the impact of the intervention. As suggested by Williamson and colleagues (1977), multiple strategies may be necessary because "it is difficult to find the single procedure which will produce the initial verbal response in the nonverbal environment" (p. 143).

Thus far, strict operant and behavioral approaches (i.e., positive reinforcement) have been combined with stimulus fading procedures (e.g., Conrad et al. 1974, Reid et al. 1967, Richards and Hansen 1978, Williamson et al. 1977, Wulbert et al. 1973) and family therapy techniques (Lazarus et al. 1983, Rosenberg and Lindblad 1978) with some success. Although behavioral approaches may be more effective and time-efficient than psychodynamic approaches (Kratochwill et al. 1979, Lazarus et al. 1983, Wright et al. 1985), some authors have also reported that, when employed alone, behavioral approaches such as contingency management or punishment techniques are not effective unless they are combined with other treatment strategies (e.g., Wulbert et al. 1973). Interestingly, what appear to be the two most effective techniques for treating elective mutism have not been combined into a single treatment strategy. That is, stimulus fading and, more recently, self-modeling have both proven successful in several reports of treatment outcome. This chapter reports on the combined application of these two treatment techniques with a 6-year-old elective mute girl.

TREATMENT TECHNIQUES

STIMULUS FADING

Stimulus fading has been described in the mutism literature as a treatment technique that involves changing the stimuli that control speech "so that over time, a larger number of situations become discriminative stimuli for speaking" (Labbe and Williamson 1984, p. 277). Typically, the treatment begins in a situation where the child will readily respond verbally and then progresses gradually to situations which successively approximate the setting where speech is least likely to occur (Conrad et al. 1974). Stimuli from the "safe" environment are gradually faded out as stimuli from the more threatening situations are gradually faded in (Labbe and Williamson 1984, Richards and Hansen 1978). Assuming that the child is not speaking in the school environment, therapists employing stimulus fading will often begin treatment either in the home environment with the mother present (Conrad et al. 1974, Richards and Hansen 1978), at a clinic (Reid et al. 1967, Williamson et al. 1977, Wulbert et al. 1973), or in a "safe" location within the school (Lipton 1980, Rosenbaum and Kellman 1973). Aspects of the classroom environment (e.g., teacher, classmates, environmental cues) are then gradually introduced with the expectation that the child will produce the desired verbal behavior for each new stimulus before moving to a more difficult stimulus.

It is important to note that this definition of stimulus fading is not in line with the definition most often used in the behavior modification literature. For example, Kazdin (1977) defines *fading* as "the gradual removal of a prompt" (p. 15). That is, stimulus fading involves the gradual removal of a stimulus that has previously served to initiate a desired response. If a child with elective mutism is able to talk at home but refuses to talk at school, a "true" stimulus fading treatment would involve only the gradual removal of home stimuli. The purpose of introducing school-related stimuli (in addition to the fading out of home stimuli) is to expand the range of stimulus control to include situations other than the home environment in the child's speaking repertoire. This second component of the treatment is more properly referred to as stimulus generalization or transfer of training (Kazdin 1977, also see Kratochwill et al. 1979). To be in line with the current literature, we will continue to refer to this "fading out/fading in" procedure as stimulus fading, despite the fact that this type of treatment includes both stimulus fading and generalization components.

It is also critical to note that this strategy differs from other behavioral techniques such as shaping and in vivo desensitization.

Stimulus fading is useful when a child is already able to exhibit the desired behavior, but not in all situations. Shaping would be employed if the desired behavior has not yet occurred in any setting and the therapist rewards successive approximations to the desired behavior. Conrad et al. (1974) described the difference between these two techniques in the following manner: stimulus fading "involved bringing responses already in the child's repertoire under new stimulus control, and was not a case of shaping new behaviors which were lacking in the child's repertoire" (p. 99).

In the present instance, treatment was begun at the clinic and speech was established with the child's parents before introducing the therapist and, later, the child's teacher and two classmates. Therapy was then moved to the school where speech was again established with a parent in a neutral location, followed by the introduction of classmates and the teacher in the classroom environment.

SELF-MODELING

Self-modeling is a relatively new technique that involves "the behavioral change that results from the repeated observation of oneself on videotapes that show only desired target behaviors" (Dowrick and Dove 1980, p. 51). In the three studies using this technique with elective mute children (i.e., Dowrick and Hood 1978, Kehle et al. 1990, Pigott and Gonzales 1987, although see Bednar 1974, and Colligan et al. 1977, for examples involving audiotape self-monitoring), the child's responses to maternal questions were combined via editing procedures with the same questions by the teacher. In other words, although the electively mute children initially responded to their mothers' questions, it appeared on the tape as if the children were responding to the teacher. The child is then able to review the tape at home or, as was done in one study (Kehle et al. 1990), in front of the entire class.

The advantages of this technique are many (Pigott and Gonzales 1987): (1) most children like seeing themselves on television, thus making this treatment strategy enjoyable; (2) self-modeling appears to increase a child's feeling of self-efficacy in the area of difficulty (also see Kehle et al. 1990); (3) modeling often has a disinhibiting effect on behavior (Bandura 1969); (4) less time may be required of the therapist, given that videotapes can be viewed in one's home; and (5) there is no more appropriate model than oneself, given findings that the most appropriate models are those that are most similar to the subject. Self-modeling is especially appropriate for this population, given that peer modeling is experienced by these children on a daily basis but with no ensuing change in behavior (Kehle et al. 1990).

COMBINING TREATMENT TECHNIQUES

Given the potential advantages of each of these approaches, it seemed likely that a combination of the two may be particularly beneficial. With the case discussed in this report, a modified form of self-modeling was employed. Rather than using videotape editing procedures, which requires a degree of technical expertise as well as time, each stage of the stimulus fading procedure was videotaped and each successful verbalization from the child was shown to the child prior to beginning the next (more difficult) stage of the stimulus fading procedure. In this way, the stimulus fading and self-modeling procedures were truly integrated into a single treatment approach. Moreover, because the child enjoyed viewing herself on the television, the self-modeling procedure also served as a positive reinforcer at each stage of treatment.

CASE ILLUSTRATION

IDENTIFYING INFORMATION AND HISTORY OF PRESENTING PROBLEMS

At the time of her first appointment, Mary was a 6-year, 4-month-old Filipino girl who was in the first grade at a parochial school. She lived with her natural mother (38 years old), natural father (45 years old), brother (11 years old), and sister (12 years old). All three children were attending the same school. Mary's parents emigrated from the Philippines to the United States about fifteen years prior to treatment. English was the first language of all three children and the second language of the parents. Both parents were employed in science-related fields.

Mary was brought to the outpatient child psychiatry clinic because she would not talk in school. Her parents were also concerned about two episodes where Mary "froze up" during a piano recital. Mary had not talked to her teacher or any of her classmates in school during her one-and-a-half years at the school. She also would not answer the phone or talk to people she did not know (e.g., store clerks, mailmen, etc.). On the other hand, she would talk to all members of her family (including cousins, uncles, and aunts) and family friends. She had not been enrolled in a preschool, day-care program, or church school, and all babysitters were family members (e.g., grandmother and cousins). Thus, it was only when Mary began school that her parents became aware of the severity of her problem.

Prior to treatment, Mary's teachers had employed a number of strategies to address her lack of speech. For example, her kindergarten teacher instructed her to stand in the back of the room when she would not talk. Unfortunately, a few days after this strategy was implemented, Mary began crying in the middle of the night, developed diurnal enuresis, and began coming home from school complaining of stomachaches. Although Mary's first-grade teacher also used isolation, she reported that she eventually began ignoring the problem because Mary was capable of doing her schoolwork when given verbal instructions. In an attempt to help Mary talk to her kindergarten teacher, Mary's parents invited the teacher to dinner at their home. During this visit, Mary talked to her brother and sister in front of the teacher but never addressed the teacher directly. Mary's parents also tried a variety of rewards (e.g., clothes, dolls) and punishments (e.g., spanking), none of which were helpful.

Mary's parents discussed a number of other events that appeared to be potentially related to the development of the mutism. When Mary was nearly 2 years old, her family took a one-month trip to the Philippines to visit relatives. Throughout this trip, Mary insisted on having her mother at her side at all times. When she was 4 years old, Mary began taking piano lessons and was able to talk to the teacher (whom she knew prior to taking lessons), but only if some family member (e.g., mother, brother, or sister) was also present. Subsequently, she was asked to perform in two piano recitals in front of approximately forty people. On both occasions, she went to the recital, walked across the stage to the piano, but then refused to play.

DEVELOPMENTAL, EDUCATIONAL, AND FAMILY HISTORY

Mary was the 6 lb., 1 oz. product of an unplanned, full-term pregnancy with no complications. No feeding or sleep problems were noted. She crawled at 5 months, walked at 12 months, talked at 1½ years, and used words with meaning at 2 years. Urinary and bowel control were reportedly established at 18 months. All of her school evaluations were positive except in the area of language development. On the Clymer-Barrett Readiness Test (administered at school), she performed at the 95th percentile across all subject areas (i.e., visual discrimination, auditory discrimination, and visual-motor coordination).

Both of Mary's parents came to the United States "to look for adventure, a good job, and more money." They met and got married shortly after arriving in this country. Mary's father moved here with his mother and stayed with two sisters. He was the third child of five (he had two brothers and two sisters). Although his mother was still living, his father died in 1967. Mary's mother came from a large family (nine siblings); her mother lived in the Philippines and her father died in 1973. Although Mary's mother's parents were both nonprofessionals (e.g., her father only reached the fourth grade), they felt that education for their children was "the highest priority" and that their "ambition in life" was to have their children become professionals. Similarly, Mary's father's parents were both nonprofessionals and they too placed a high value on education.

ASSESSMENT DATA

On the Parent Temperament Questionnaire for Children (Thomas and Chess 1977), Mary's parents described her as demonstrating positive mood but a tendency to withdraw socially and have a low threshold for changes in her environment. When Mary's parents were asked to describe early temperamental differences between their children, they described both daughters as "shy and dependent." On the Achenbach Child Behavior Checklist (Achenbach and Edelbrock 1983), Mary was reported (by her mother) to have clinically significant levels (i.e., above the 98th percentile) on the following scales: Social Withdrawal, Schizoid-Obsessive, Depression, and the overall Internalizing Scale. At the item level. Mary was reported to be shy and timid but also very stubborn. The shyness was apparently situational because Mary's mother also reported that she talks too much at home. Mary's father tended to endorse fewer items than did her mother; none of the scales were significantly elevated for father's report. On the teacher version of the Achenbach Child Behavior Checklist, Mary's teacher reported significant elevations on the Anxious and the overall Internalizing scales. At the item level, her teacher reported that she was nervous, shy, stubborn, clingy to adults, and feared that she would not perform well in school.

FORMULATION

Although the causes of Mary's difficulties are not known, it appears that the mutism resulted from a number of contributing factors. Both her teacher and parents reported that Mary was a temperamentally shy and timid girl—behaviors that seemed to be most apparent when she was in an unfamiliar environment. She also appeared to have had a moderately symbiotic relationship with her mother where clinginess was reinforced since very early in Mary's life. Mary's mother appeared to be very sensitive to her distress and responded by being protective of her. As a result, Mary received considerable amounts of attention for her problem and the reinforcement (secondary gain) may have exacerbated her shyness.

Mary's parents also had high achievement expectations for themselves and their children, expectations that may have increased Mary's performance anxiety. As a consequence, the avoidance of talking was negatively reinforced by the decrease in anxiety. Moreover, by not talking, Mary may not have been required to meet all of her parents' expectations. Talking brings with it a set of responsibilities that may have been undesirable to Mary. Finally, Mary was (according to her mother and her teacher) a very stubborn child who enjoyed being in control of her environment. Interestingly, some have reported that elective mutes are often sensitive to being controlled (Lesser-Katz 1988). It was expected, therefore, that Mary would stubbornly hold on to her symptoms if the benefits outweighed the costs.

TREATMENT AND OUTCOME

Treatment was begun after two diagnostic interviews with the entire family. Mary did not speak during the first meeting, but did give adequate amounts of eye contact. She was observed to be quite clingy to her parents while walking down the hall to the meeting room and frequently sat on her mother's or father's lap. In the second session, she answered questions but would do so by whispering her answers into her mother's ear. At the end of both of these initial diagnostic sessions, Mary separated easily from her parents to engage in free play with the therapist, which usually consisted of simple drawing and writing tasks.

As is often done at the beginning of treatment with an elective mute (e.g., Lipton 1980), initiation of speech with the therapist was shaped by first requiring Mary to blow a piece of paper across a desk, the notion being that this type of mouth activity would make her more comfortable with other more anxiety-provoking speech behaviors. Unfortunately, Mary refused (for three sessions) to participate in this type of activity, despite being offered rewards such as candy, cartoon stickers, or praise. Because little progress was made in these play sessions, a different strategy was implemented. Beginning with session 6, Mary and her parents were brought to a room where they could be videotaped. They were instructed to interact verbally around a drawing task while the therapist observed behind a two-way mirror. With much hesitation at first, Mary talked with her parents, but only when the therapist was absent from the room.

Given that Mary had now begun to speak aloud at the clinic, the stimulus fading/self-modeling procedure was initiated in sessions 7 and 8. Mary and her parents were again instructed to talk in the observation room. After conversation was established, the father was asked to leave the room (to run the video camera) and the mother was asked to stand by the door of the room, but still within sight of her daughter. So as to give Mary a sense of control (Lesser-Katz 1988), Mary was asked to position the therapist at a point in the hallway (outside of the room) where she would still be comfortable talking aloud to her mother but where the therapist could also overhear her conversation. Mary was then instructed to return to the observation room and continue her conversation with her mother. Once the conversation was reestablished, Mary, her parents, and the therapist viewed a video replay of the conversation that had just occurred between Mary and her mother. In this way, Mary and the therapist could observe Mary and her mother talking; it was expected that this experience would make her more likely to initiate conversation with the therapist. Several of these stimulus fading/self-modeling sequences were conducted with the mother eventually being moved out of the room and the therapist gradually being introduced into the room (i.e., standing in the back of the room with back toward Mary, sitting in a chair close to Mary but with face hidden, etc.). After talking was established at each step, videotape feedback was employed both as a self-modeling technique and as a reinforcer. By the end of session 7, Mary was able to recite the alphabet to the therapist while maintaining eye contact. After session 8, she was able to talk freely to the therapist.

Generalization to the school environment was begun at the clinic in session 9. Mary's best friend and classmate (Kate) was brought to the clinic and again the stimulus fading/self-modeling procedure was employed with success (see Conrad et al. 1974). By the end of the session, she talked freely and with much enthusiasm with her friend. Prior to this session, Mary had never talked to Kate, despite requests by the therapist that they get together at Mary's house to talk. During the next week, Mary's teacher reported that Mary whispered to Kate in class. She also talked to Kate on the phone on several occasions after this session. In session 10, the therapist talked with Mary in various areas of the clinic and the adjoining hospital (e.g., the cafeteria). In session 11, Kate and another student from Mary's class (Kathy) were brought in and, after applying the fading/modeling procedure, Mary talked freely with both students. She also met with a psychiatrist on the same day as this session and she talked freely with him with little fading or modeling required.

Finally, Mary's teacher was brought into the clinic (session 12) and the same fading/modeling procedure was employed. Because Mary talked to her teacher during this session, it was decided that during the next school day the therapist would begin treatment in the school setting. At this point in the treatment process, only the stimulus fading procedure was employed owing to the intrusiveness of the self-modeling procedure. During the first school visit, Mary talked to her teacher, a school administrator, and several students (all individually). Subsequently, Mary's teacher reported that Mary whispered to her during class time but would not speak out loud. On three subsequent visits to the school, and in order to more closely approximate the nature of the classroom environment, Mary was asked to talk aloud to peers in groups of three to four both outside and (later) inside the classroom. Although this strategy was successful, it was observed that she had more difficulty speaking out loud in the classroom than outside the classroom.

In order to maintain the progress Mary already made and generalize her skills to other aspects of the classroom environment, a contingency management system was employed in place of the fading procedure (see Labbe and Williamson 1984, Richards and Hansen 1978). Mary was instructed to stand halfway between her desk and the teacher's desk during roll call and whisper "here." She also had to whisper at least one word during reading group. If she performed satisfactorily, she would receive cartoon stickers on a daily basis that could be traded for a new coloring book. After repeated successes, the tasks were made more difficult (e.g., Mary had to whisper from her desk during roll call and whisper five words in reading group). By the end of the school year, Mary was consistently whispering in all classroom settings (e.g., she could read passages from a book in reading group) and speaking aloud on some occasions. In addition to talking at school, Mary also became more involved with her peers. She reportedly talked aloud at birthday parties and continued to talk aloud to several of her friends at school.

At six-month follow-up (middle of second grade), Mary's mother reported that she was talking freely to her classroom and physical education teachers and several of her classmates, and was talking aloud in reading group. Her mother also reported that she had performed successfully in two piano recitals at the beginning of second grade. On the other hand, she was still uncomfortable talking aloud to the entire class; her teacher reported that she would still whisper when in a large group setting.

CONCLUSION

As demonstrated by the case study, it appears that stimulus fading and self-modeling can be combined into a successful single treatment strategy for elective mutism. Mary began speaking in clinic and school settings after seven clinic sessions involving the fading and modeling procedure and four school consultation visits. In past case studies that have employed self-modeling (Dowrick and Hood 1978, Kehle et al. 1990, Pigott and Gonzales 1987), tape editing techniques were required to make it appear as if the child was speaking in situations where the child was ordinarily silent (e.g., the school classroom). Unlike these earlier approaches, unedited videotape feedback was provided to Mary after each successful step of the stimulus fading procedure. In this way, the feedback served both as a self-modeling technique and as a positive reinforcer for a child who enjoyed seeing herself on television. The results of this case also demonstrated the utility of contingency management approaches in bridging the gap between clinic and school settings (Richards and Hansen 1978).

Although the techniques described here were successful, it is important to note that this child was still reluctant to verbalize aloud in some group settings (e.g., in front of the entire class). In previous studies, a number of investigators have reported that electively mute children tend to be shy, even after treatment has been applied (e.g., Bednar 1974, Conrad et al. 1974, Lesser-Katz 1988). Given the consistency of these findings, it is likely that elective mutism occurs in children who are temperamentally predisposed to be shy, socially withdrawn, and emotionally subdued (Jones et al. 1986, Kagan 1989). In fact, there appears to be considerable longitudinal behavioral continuity with respect to such behaviors; Kagan (1989) has found that roughly 75 percent of children who were classified as inhibited at age 2 or 3 were still classified as inhibited at age 7½ years. Thus, it is not surprising that Mary continued to be somewhat inhibited, despite the application of several sessions of effective treatments. It is likely that Mary will need counseling periodically throughout her childhood and adolescence. Changes in schools and increasing peer and educational demands may be stressful for Mary and she may need psychological services at these particular developmental transition points (Holmbeck and Kendall 1991).

The continuity issue aside, we would still maintain, as have others (e.g., Wright et al. 1985), that the long-term prognosis for children with elective mutism is likely to improve with early identification and intervention. Unfortunately, there is often a lag of two to three years between age of onset (i.e., during the preschool years) and age of referral (in kindergarten or first grade; Wright et al. 1985). It is only through education efforts directed to pediatricians and preschool teachers that the symptoms of electively mute children can be addressed soon after the difficulties are evident.

REFERENCES

Achenbach, T. M., and Edelbrock, C. S. (1983). *Manual for the Child Behavior Checklist and Revised Child Behavior Profile.* Burlington: University of Vermont.

Albert-Stewart, P. L. (1986). Positive reinforcement in short-term treatment of an electively mute child: a case study. *Psychological Reports* 58:571–576.

American Psychiatric Association. (1987). *Diagnostic and Statistical Manual of Mental Disorders, Third Edition, Revised (DSM-III-R).* Washington, DC: American Psychiatric Association.

Atoynatan, T. H. (1986). Elective mutism: involvement of the mother in the treatment of the child. *Child Psychiatry and Human Development* 17:15–27.

Bandura, A. (1969). *Principles of Behavior Modification.* New York: Holt, Rinehart, and Winston.

Barlow, K., Strother, J., and Landreth, G. (1986). Sibling group play therapy: an effective alternative with an elective mute child. *School Counselor* 34:44–50.

Bednar, R. A. (1974). A behavioral approach to treating an elective mute in the school. *Journal of School Psychology* 12:326–337.

Chethik, M. (1973). The intensive treatment of an elective mute. *Journal of the American Academy of Child Psychiatry* 12:482–498.

Colligan, R. W., Colligan, R. C., and Dilliard, M. K. (1977). Contingency management in the classroom treatment of long-term elective mutism: a case report. *Journal of School Psychology* 15:9–17.

Conrad, R. D., Delk, J. L., and Williams, C. (1974). Use of stimulus fading procedures in the treatment of situation specific mutism: a case study. *Journal of Behavior Therapy and Experimental Psychiatry* 5:99–100.

Dowrick, P. W., and Dove, C. (1980). The use of self-modeling to improve the swimming performance of spina bifida children. *Journal of Applied Behavior Analysis* 13:51–56.

Dowrick, P. W., and Hood, M. (1978). Transfer of talking behavior across settings using faked films. In *Proceedings of the New Zealand Conference for Research in Applied Behavior Analysis,* ed. E. L. Glynn and S. S. McNaughton. Auckland, New Zealand: University of Auckland Press.

Hayden, T. L. (1980). Classification of elective mutism. *Journal of the American Academy of Child Psychiatry* 19:118–133.

Hoffman, S., and Laub, B. (1986). Paradoxical intervention using a polarization model of cotherapy in the treatment of elective mutism: a case study. *Contemporary Family Therapy* 8:136–143.

Holmbeck, G. N., and Kendall, P. (1991). Clinical-childhood-developmental interface: Implications for treatment. In *Handbook of Behavior Therapy and Psychological Science: An Integrative Approach*, ed. P. R. Martin, pp. 73–99. New York: Pergamon.

Jones, W. H., Cheek, J. M., and Briggs, S. R., eds. (1986). *Shyness: Perspectives on Research and Treatment.* New York: Plenum.

Kagan, J. (1989). Temperamental contributions to social behavior. *American Psychologist* 44:668–674.

Kazdin, A. E. (1977). *The Token Economy: A Review and Evaluation.* New York: Plenum.

Kehle, T. J., Owen, S. V., and Cressy, E. T. (1990). The use of self-modeling as an intervention in school psychology: a case study of an elective mute. *School Psychology Review* 19:115–121.

Kolvin, I., and Fundudis, T. (1981). Elective mute children: psychological development and background factors. *Journal of Child Psychology and Psychiatry* 22:219–232.

Kratochwill, T. R., Brody, G. H., and Piersel, W. C. (1979). Elective mutism in children. In *Advances in Clinical Child Psychology*, vol. 2, ed. B. B. Lahey and A. E. Kazdin, pp. 193–240. New York: Plenum.

Labbe, E. E., and Williamson, D. A. (1984). Behavioral treatment of elective mutism: a review of the literature. *Clinical Psychology Review* 4:273–292.

Lazarus, P. J., Gavilo, H. M., and Moore, J. W. (1983). The treatment of elective mutism in children within the school setting: two case studies. *School Psychology Review* 12:467–472.

Lesser-Katz, M. (1986). Stranger reaction and elective mutism in young children. *American Journal of Orthopsychiatry* 56:458–469.

——— (1988). The treatment of elective mutism as stranger reaction. *Psychotherapy* 25:305–313.

Lipton, H. (1980). Rapid reinstatement of speech using stimulus fading with a selectively mute child. *Journal of Behavior Therapy and Experimental Psychiatry* 11:147–149.

Meyers, S. V. (1984). Elective mutism in children: a family systems approach. *American Journal of Family Therapy* 12:39–45.

Morin, C., Ladouceur, R., and Cloutier, R. (1982). Reinforcement procedure in the treatment of reluctant speech. *Journal of Behavior Therapy and Experimental Psychiatry* 13:145–147.

Nash, R. T., Thorpe, H. W., Andrews, M. M., and Davis, K. (1979). A management program for elective mutism. *Psychology in the Schools* 16:246–253.

Nolan, J. D., and Pence, C. (1970). Operant conditioning principles in the treatment of a selectively mute child. *Journal of Consulting and Clinical Psychology* 35:265–268.

Pigott, H. E., and Gonzales, F. P. (1987). Efficacy of videotape self-modeling in treating an electively mute child. *Journal of Clinical Child Psychology* 16:106–110.

Reid, J. R., Hawkins, N., Keutzer, C., et al. (1967). A marathon behavior modification of a selectively mute child. *Journal of Child Psychology and Psychiatry* 8:27–30.

Richards, C. S., and Hansen, M. K. (1978). A further demonstration of the efficacy of stimulus fading treatment of elective mutism. *Journal of Behavior Therapy and Experiental Psychiatry* 9:57–60.

Rosenbaum, E., and Kellman, M. (1973). Treatment of a selectively mute third-grade child. *Journal of School Psychology* 11:26–29.

Rosenberg, J. B., and Lindblad, M. B. (1978). Behavior therapy in a family context: treating elective mutism. *Family Process* 17:77–82.

Rutter, M., and Garmezy, N. (1983). Developmental psychopathology. In *Handbook of Child Psychology, Vol. 4: Socialization, Personality, and Social Development*, ed. E. M. Hetherington and P. H. Mussen, series ed., pp. 775–911. New York: Wiley.

Sanok, R. L., and Striefel, S. (1979). Elective mutism: generalization of verbal responding across people and settings. *Behavior Therapy* 10:357–371.

Thomas, A., and Chess, S. (1977). *Temperament and Development*. New York: Brunner/Mazel.

van der Kooy, D., and Webster, C. D. (1975). A rapidly effective behavior modification program for an electively mute child. *Journal of Behavior Therapy and Experimental Psychiatry* 6:149–152.

Wergeland, H. (1979). Elective mutism. *Acta Psychiatrica Scandinavica* 59:218–228.

Wilkins, R. (1985). A comparison of elective mutism and emotional disorders in children. *British Journal of Psychiatry* 146:198–203.

Williamson, D. A., Sanders, S. H., Sewell, W. R., et al. (1977). The behavioral treatment of elective mutism: two case studies. *Journal of Behavior Therapy and Experimental Psychiatry* 8:143–149.

Wright, H. H., Miller, D., Cook, M. A., and Littmann, J. R. (1985). Early identification and intervention with children who refuse to speak. *Journal of the American Academy of Child Psychiatry* 24:739–746.

Wulbert, M., Nyman, B. A., Snow, D., and Owen, Y. (1973). The efficacy of stimulus fading and contingency management in the treatment of elective mutism: a case study. *Journal of Applied Behavior Analysis* 6:435–441.

7

AN ADAPTED LANGUAGE TRAINING STRATEGY IN THE TREATMENT OF AN ELECTIVELY MUTE MALE CHILD

Edward V. Pecukonis and Marya T. Pecukonis

RESEARCH HAS DOCUMENTED the usefulness of behavioral procedures in the acquisition and remediation of verbal language (Harris 1975). Clearly, the absence of verbal language is a debilitating and limiting deficit, which often results in progressive social and emotional isolation (Berrera et al. 1980, Krolian 1988).

In general, language training strategies have been employed with subjects displaying severe deficits in spoken language skills. However, few studies have attempted to adapt these models of language training to the treatment of subjects who possess sufficient verbal repertoires but have difficulty in either identifying the discriminative stimuli for speech, or are unable to embrace the self-reinforcing value of interpersonal communication (Sherman 1965).

Within the professional literature these individuals are typically identified by the ambiguous label *elective mutism* (Isaacs et al. 1965). This sweeping diagnostic class appears to encompass a wide range of language deficits including selective or situational speech refusal, and extreme verbal response latencies. Although the child has the ability to comprehend spoken language, speech is avoided in almost all social situations (Louden 1987). Age of onset is typically between 3 and 5 years and is associated with the child entering school.

Considering the extensive research that has been directed at developing basic verbal skills in nonverbal subjects, it is surprising that research has neglected the opportunity to adapt these conditioning strategies for modifying elective mutism. Thus, this chapter constructs an adapted language training strategy for ameliorating elective mutism.

LANGUAGE TRAINING MODELS

Recently, research using verbal conditioning has focused on developing effective expressive language training strategies. These studies have appeared in the literature under such diverse headings as mediated language acquisition (Gray 1968), programmed communication training (Marshall and Hegrenes 1970), language development training (Bloom 1970, Bricker and Bricker 1970), linguistic competence (Fygetakis 1970), and establishing imitative speech (Borus 1973), and have been used with autistic children (Evans 1971), aphasic children (Blake and Moss 1967), echolalic children (Risley and Wolf 1967), and the intellectually handicapped (Baer and Guess 1971, Garcia 1974). Most of these training strategies consist of four basic steps: (1) attention training, (2) nonverbal imitation, (3) verbal imitation, and (4) functional language training.

NONVERBAL ATTENDING

An important prerequisite for facilitating speech lies in gaining the attention of the subject. Typical interventions have employed shaping with positive reinforcement to establish eye contact with the subject (Kozloff 1973). Brooks and colleagues (1968) encouraged the establishment of eye contact with the verbal prompt "Look at me," initially reinforced on a continuous fixed ratio basis, using primary reinforcement paired with social praise. Contingencies were later modified to a variable ratio schedule as response criteria were met.

The development of attending behaviors in electively mute subjects is important since these individuals avoid verbal interaction in social situations through withdrawal, shyness and negativism (*DSM-III-R*; American Psychiatric Association 1987). These behaviors may interfere with their ability to attend to the conversational cues in their environment.

NONVERBAL AND VERBAL IMITATION

In nonverbal imitative behavior training the subject is taught a series of gross motor behaviors such as clapping, standing, and touching one's toes that are gradually shaped through successive approximations to specific facial movements instrumental in producing speech (Bricker and Bricker 1970). Unfortunately, it is debatable whether nonverbal imitation training either accentuates or facilitates generalization to later verbal imitative training (Garcia et al. 1971, Harris 1975).

Since electively mute individuals possess sufficient skills in language comprehension and fluency, training in nonverbal imitative behaviors appears contraindicated and superfluous. However, training strategies should focus on increasing verbal imitative behaviors. Lovaas and colleagues (1966) have outlined a generic strategy of verbal imitative training employing four basic steps: (1) rewarding all vocalizations, (2) rewarding vocalization occurring within six seconds of the models vocalization, (3) rewarding vocalization within six seconds of the models vocalizations that successively approximates the vocalization of the model, and (4) the introduction of novel vocalizations by the model, beginning at step three.

FUNCTIONAL LANGUAGE

The main emphasis of language training has been the development of functional language. Subjects are typically taught noun labels first and then other forms of grammar (Baer 1968, Guess 1969). Functional language training emphasizes conversation skills and generalization of these abilities across situations, settings, and persons beyond the treatment room. This phase of traditional language training is particularly relevant to the initiation of conversational speech for the electively mute individual. In many ways, an electively mute child has difficulty in discriminating the appropriate cues encouraging verbal interactions. Thus, the subject is unable to elicit the normal social reinforcing events that encourage and maintain verbal interaction with others.

Barton (1972) attempted to encourage conversational speech in an electively mute subject using a multiple baseline across behaviors design. He found that subjects increased their conversational speech with the delivery of secondary reinforcers in the form of tokens. It was shown that tokens were significantly more effective at reducing response latencies than the direct administration of primary reinforcers. In a later study with a group of electively mute subjects Barton (1975) administered tokens for appropriate verbal communication. At the end of the 15-minute session, tokens were counted and an assortment of items (sweets, cigarettes, tea, coffee, and trinkets) were displayed at varying costs. The prizes were then given to the subjects with an explanation as to why they were receiving these rewards. The rate of conversational speech improved significantly. However, generalization to other situations was minimal.

Clearly, problems of generalization have been characteristic of language training programs (Koegel and Rincover 1974). Garcia (1974) stressed the importance of using more than one trainer during language acquisition training to improve generalization of behaviors. Kazdin and Bootzin (1972) state that generalization usually is not obtained unless it is programmed as part of the procedure. Their suggestions are (1) remove reinforcement gradually, (2) alter the schedules of reinforcement once acquisition of the response has taken place, (3) alter the environment, (4) involve family and relatives in implementing contingencies, and (5) establish a delay period in both earning and exchanging tokens.

In summary, it would appear that an effective language training program for electively mute individuals can be adapted from training strategies used with nonverbal subjects. As outlined above, useful program strategies would include (1) attention training, (2) imitative and functional language training, and (3) procedures geared to encourage generalization across situations and persons. Language training research has also documented the usefulness of both primary and secondary positive reinforcers in combination with shaping procedures, prompts, and social praise in the establishment of functional language. Therapeutic change is best documented across phases of training employing a multiple baseline across behaviors experimental design.

METHOD

SUBJECT

A 7-year-old African-American boy served as the subject for the present study. The child was the youngest of an intact family, consisting of his parents and two older brothers who reside in a rural area. The child attended a local special education program for handicapped children.

Developmentally, the child was delayed in negotiating many major milestones (e.g., rolling over, walking, speech, etc.). At 2 years of age the child's parents were concerned about his general lack of affect and interest in the people and objects around him. At age 5 the child was referred by his family physician for a comprehensive evaluation. At the time of this referral he was seen by a neurologist and psychologist. This evaluation revealed a moderate intellectual limitation with significant depressive features. His full scale I.Q. was measured at 63 on the Wechsler Intelligence Scale for Children, Revised (WISC-R) with minimal variability between verbal and performance subscales.

Although the subject had developed appropriate speech consistent with his intellectual abilities, he became socially withdrawn, reticent, and at times negativistic. After he entered school, these behaviors continued to deteriorate and by age 7 the subject began to exhibit marked verbal inhibition and was diagnosed as being electively mute. The child refused to speak in almost all social situations, despite excellent receptive language skills. The child's speech was characterized by extreme response latencies, terse utterances (often monosyllabic), and impaired nonverbal attending skills. Verbal interaction was limited to his family.

BASELINE

This early phase allowed for an adaptation to the treatment environment and the selection of edible reinforcers. Baseline measures were taken across the target behaviors of (1) nonverbal attending, (2) verbal imitative behavior, and (3) functional language abilities. Each 45-minute observational period was broken into three 15-minute blocks. Each of these 15-minute blocks was dedicated to assessing one of the three behaviors in question.

Nonverbal attending was assessed as the percentage of appropriate responses (making eye contact with the experimenter) to the request "Look at me." This request was made every sixty seconds for a total of fifteen requests during a 15-minute observation period.

A list of fifteen nouns representing familiar and important objects from the child's environment was constructed and used to measure imitative language. During this 15-minute block, the nouns were identified verbally by the trainer. Following each word presentation, the trainer asked the child to repeat the word.

Assessment of functional language incorporated the development of a list of thirty open-ended questions generated from the fifteen-item noun list (two questions per noun). Prior to each session fifteen questions were randomly selected in such a manner that each of the fifteen nouns was represented.

A reinforcement menu was constructed through detailed interviews with the child's teachers and parents. Spontaneous verbal interaction outside of the treatment session was also monitored at school by the child's classroom teacher and at home by his parents.

Any intelligible verbal utterances were counted. This monitoring occurred throughout all phases of training and was used to ascertain the effects of generalization.

TRAINING NONVERBAL ATTENDING

The training of nonverbal attending behaviors was implemented in this phase of the study. This component skill was operationally defined as the child's ability to make eye contact with the trainer(s) within five seconds of the verbal prompt, "Look at me." If the child fixated visually (attended) to the trainer within five seconds of his verbal request, the subject was positively reinforced with verbal praise and a token that could either be saved or cashed in for backup (primary) reinforcers at the completion of the training session (e.g., consumables such as candy, cookies, or snack cakes). Nickels were used as tokens.

To expedite acquisition during this training phase the child's parents were also involved in the training and provided additional social praise and physical prompts (e.g., turning the subject's head toward the trainer). Training continued until a level of 90 percent appropriate attending behavior was reached and maintained for four successive training sessions (i.e., making eye contact with the trainer within five seconds of her request). During this stage of acquisition, tokens and praise were delivered on a continuous, fixed ratio schedule (FR 1).

TRAINING VERBAL IMITATION

As noted previously prior to training, a list of fifteen nouns representing familiar and important objects from the subject's environment was developed. This list was constructed with the aid of the subject's teachers and parents, and was used during both baseline and treatment phases. The nouns selected are listed in Table 7-1.

During this phase of training each of the fifteen nouns was identified verbally by the trainer while holding the object in clear view of the subject. For example, as a baseball was presented visually, the

Table 7–1.
Noun Words Used for Verbal Imitative Responding

(1) bike (photo)	(6) record (Beat It)	(11) Walkie Talkie
(2) dog (photo)	(7) toy gun	(12) puppet
(3) baseball	(8) game	(13) Star Wars man
(4) baseball glove	(9) dump truck	(14) animal poster
(5) Orioles hat	(10) basketball	(15) puzzle

trainer stated, "This is a baseball." "Say baseball." Verbal imitative behavior was operationally defined as being appropriate if (1) the child made eye contact with the trainer, (2) verbally imitated the noun word presented within five seconds of the trainer's request, and (3) the verbal production was audible and recognizable. If the response was appropriate, the object was given to the child with a token and verbal praise. If no response occurred within thirty seconds, the next item on the list was presented. This procedure continued until all fifteen items were presented.

Tokens and praise were presented on a continuous schedule until a criterion of 90 percent appropriate responding was met during two successive training sessions. Following the end of each training session, the child was allowed to exchange his tokens for consumables or the option of keeping any of the objects presented until the next training session.

A new contingency was added during this training phase. The child was informed that he could purchase a wristwatch if he saved enough tokens. This contingency would (1) encourage a temporal delay between appropriate responding and actual reinforcement, (2) prevent reinforcement satiation, and (3) increase motivation during the next phase of training. To promote generalization, the parents and trainer took turns in presenting the objects/noun words to the subject. All verbal and physical prompts for nonverbal attending behavior were faded out by the completion of this phase of training.

FUNCTIONAL CONVERSATION

Functional language training was directed at establishing functional conversational skills. During this phase of training a list of thirty open-ended questions were generated from the fifteen-item noun list (two questions per word). These thirty questions are listed in Table 7-2.

Prior to each training session fifteen questions were randomly selected in such a fashion that each of the fifteen nouns was represented. Thus, one open-ended question was asked about each object over fifteen trials. To enhance the child's motivation, puppets were used by the trainer, parents, and child during conversational interactions. During this phase the trainer held the object in his hand and posed the open-ended question to the subject using the puppet. Appropriate responses were operationally defined as follows: (1) the child fixated visually and responded verbally within five seconds of the trainer's request, (2) responses were audible and recognizable, (3) response content was consistent with the topic being discussed, and (4) responses consisted of at least a two-word sentence. The child was given the object along with a token and social praise for appropriate responses. If the subject responded with more than one sentence, he was given a bonus token. Again, reinforcement was delivered on a continuous fixed-ratio schedule. Training continued until the subject had reached a 90 percent appropriate response criterion over two successive training sessions.

GENERALIZED FUNCTIONAL VERBAL
LANGUAGE TRAINING

The final phase of treatment was directed at establishing generalized functional verbal language across persons, situations, and verbal contents. Training for generalization included (1) reinforcing appropriate verbal responses during training sessions on a variable ratio schedule of four (VR 4), (2) increasing temporal delay for "cashing in tokens" (once per week), (3) varying room settings for training, (e.g., classroom, parents' home, cafeteria, etc.), (4) allowing the child

Table 7-2.
Open-Ended Question Used for Functional Language Training

(1) What do you like about your bike?	(16) What do you do with this game?
(2) Where can you ride your bike?	(17) Can you tell me how the truck works?
(3) What do you do with your dog?	(18) How does the dirt come out?
(4) How do you take care of your dog?	(19) How do you throw the ball?
(5) What do you like about baseball?	(20) What do you like about basketball?
(6) With whom do you play baseball?	(21) How do you make the Walkie Talkie work?
(7) Why do you wear the baseball glove?	(22) What do you say into the Walkie Talkie?
(8) Can you tell me how you catch the ball?	(23) What does your puppet eat?
(9) When do you wear your Orioles hat?	(24) Can you tell me about his clothes?
(10) Why do baseball players wear hats?	(25) What can this Star Wars man do?
(11) Tell me what you like about this song.	(26) Will you tell me about his suit?
(12) Why do you like Michael Jackson's song?	(27) What does this animal feel like?
(13) Can you tell me about your gun?	(28) What does this animal eat?
(14) How does your gun work?	(29) Will you tell me how to put this puzzle together?
(15) How do you play this game?	(30) What will this puzzle make?

to earn additional tokens at home and in school between sessions for appropriate verbal responses, (5) discontinuing the use of puppets, and (6) introducing novel noun words and open-ended questions approaching normal conversation.

Recordings for verbal responding outside the treatment session was monitored by means of a tally card that the child carried on his person at all times. Teachers and family members noted each appropriate verbal interaction with a check mark, signature, and date. At the end of each week these verbal responses were tallied and cashed in for tokens. Previously outside of training session responses were recorded by teachers and parents.

In addition, each mark on the tally sheet was made contingent upon the subject asking each appropriate person to record the occurrence of verbal interactions on his tally card. This procedure was implemented with the goals of (1) increasing spontaneous speech, and (2) providing the subject with a sense of control over the positive consequences of verbal interaction.

DEPENDENT MEASURES

Discrete frequency data over four phases of adapted language training were recorded within a multiple baseline across behaviors experimental design. Training sessions were held for 45 minutes, five times per week over a six-week duration. Since baseline recordings of target behaviors were continuous, each 45-minute training session was broken into three 15-minute observational periods evaluating: (1) nonverbal attending, (2) imitative verbal responding, and (3) functional language.

The child's responses were recorded by two trained scorers during each of the 45-minute training sessions. The second scorer did not participate in the actual training but served as a reliability check on the trainer's scoring of the subject's responses. In addition, each training session was audiotaped and used as a tertiary reliability check on the accuracy of scoring. The second scorer had no influence on the delivery of reinforcement.

Assessment instruments included a stopwatch, tally sheet, and tape recorder. A response was marked on the tally sheet as appropriate or inappropriate, depending on whether it met the various criteria established during the phases of treatment. Training sessions occurred during both morning and afternoon hours. Variability in training times was employed to promote generalization, as well as to obtain an accurate sampling of behavior. During generalization of language training, recording was shifted to a quasi-continuous method since reinforcement was made available outside of the training session (e.g., home, classroom, etc.).

RELIABILITY

Response frequency data were collected across the training sessions for each of the three target behaviors over thirty-three training sessions.

Interrater reliability was computed across training sessions to ascertain the percentage of agreement between the two scorers. Interrater agreement ranged from 78 to 90 percent with the mean approximating 86 percent. The mean Kappa statistic across all phases of training approached .83, suggesting excellent error adjusted reproducibility or concordance between scorers.

RESULTS

The data for evaluating the effectiveness of the present adapted language training program are presented in Figure 7-1.

Figure 7-1 depicts the percentage of appropriate responses for nonverbal attending, verbal imitation, and functional language areas, across treatment phases and training sessions. A visual inspection of this figure suggests that training was effective at reestablishing language repertoires.

Figure 7-1 graphically depicts the baseline deficiencies as observed prior to training. Clearly, the child was unable to attend, imitate, or respond to open-ended questions, even when prompted prior to training. Appropriate responding in each of these three targeted areas was well below 20 percent.

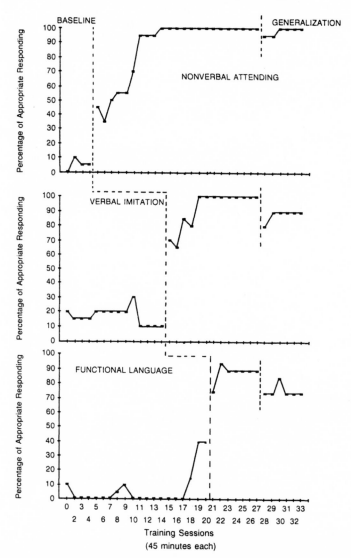

Figure 7–1. Percentage of appropriate responses for nonverbal attending, verbal imitative, and functional language responses as a function of training session

Visual attending training was initiated in session 5 with contingent reinforcement of nonverbal attending responses. As can be seen in Figure 7-1, the 90 percent response criterion was reached during session 11 and remained above criterion throughout the remainder of the treatment program. During this phase of training, baseline recordings of both verbal imitation and functional language responding was continued. Figure 7-1 notes that these responses continued to be markedly deficient and unchanged. For example, appropriate verbal imitative responses averaged 18 percent (approximately two out of fifteen words), while appropriate functional language responses occurred approximately 1 percent of the time.

The third phase of verbal imitative training was initiated during session 15, and involved the contingent reinforcement of both nonverbal attending and verbal responding by the subject to the trainer's request. Figure 7-1 notes that appropriate verbal imitative responses increased dramatically to 70 percent on the same day that reinforcement contingencies were implemented. The preestablished appropriate response criterion of 90 percent was reached during session 19 and remained at this level or above until the initiation of generalization during session 28. At this point there was a temporary decrease in imitative responses that lasted for one training session.

On the same day that the response criterion was reached for verbal imitative behavior, there was a significant increase in the appropriateness of the subject's functional language ratings, even though contingent reinforcement had not been established. On day 19 the subject's appropriate language rating reached 40 percent. Since previous ratings had been below 5 percent prior to the initiation of phase II, it may be suggested that response generalization had taken place and promoted the subject's ability to answer open-ended questions. It should be noted that on day 18 of training, the subject was informed that he could save his tokens with the goal of purchasing the wristwatch. This change in the contingencies may also help to explain the dramatic increase in functional language found during session 19.

Functional language training was initiated on day 21, and involved the contingent reinforcement of the subject attending and responding to open-ended questions posed by the trainer. The 90 percent appropriate response criterion was reached for this phase of treatment on day 22, just two sessions following its initiation. This finding also lends some support to the speculation of response generalization or carryover effect from the previous phase of training (verbal imitative).

During session 28, the fifth and final phase of language training was initiated and involved procedures aimed at promoting generalization. The data show that there was a mild decrease in appropriate responding for imitative verbal and functional language response while nonverbal attending behavior remained above criterion. Although verbal imitative behavior returned to criterion during session 29, functional language responses remained below the 90 percent criterion throughout the remainder of the training sessions. Interestingly, six sessions were necessary to reach the response criterion for nonverbal attending behavior, while only five sessions and two sessions were required for imitative verbal responding and functional language, respectively.

Finally, as the frequency of spontaneous speech was continuously recorded by both parents and teachers outside of the training sessions, the response generalization of appropriate speech across two outside settings can be evaluated.

Figure 7–2 notes the frequency of spontaneous speech at both home and school during each of the thirty-three days language training was implemented. As can be seen in Figure 7–2, the frequency of spontaneous speech at both home and school increases progressively across the thirty-three days of language training. For example, prior to initiating training, the subject exhibited zero spontaneous verbal responses at school and averaged two spontaneous verbal responses at home. During the three phases of language training the subject continued to exhibit severe spontaneous language deficits at school. However, following the initiation of generalization procedures between sessions 28 and 33, the subject averaged two to five spontaneous interactions at school. With regard to spontaneous speech at home, the subject averaged approximately four spontaneous verbal responses during the first three phases of training. This average rate

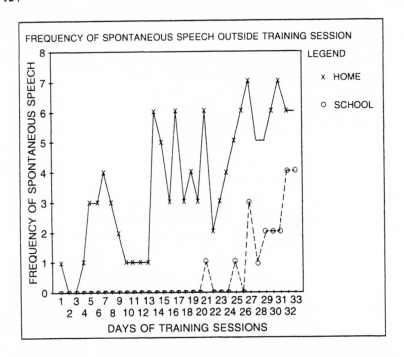

Figure 7–2. Frequency of spontaneous speech outside training session

of spontaneous speech at home increased to 5.8 responses during the generalization phase. Thus, spontaneous speech appears to have shown a progressive increase, outside of training sessions, during training for nonverbal attending, verbal attending, and functional language.

DISCUSSION

The present study investigated the usefulness of traditional language training strategies in the treatment of an electively mute 7-year-old boy. Treatment involved a variety of operant conditioning paradigms directed at improving the child's nonverbal attending skills and verbal responses to directives and questions posed by trainers. In general, the findings support the usefulness of this approach in reestablishing appropriate verbal communication. However, the present results are based on a single case, and generalizations about program effectiveness are limited. Additional research is needed to document the viability of this adapted language training program by considering subjects within various diagnostic categories and treatment settings.

The present language training model was directed at reestablishing three aspects of verbal language: (1) nonverbal attending, (2) imitative verbal responses, and (3) functional language responses. The first area of intervention was directed at improving the subject's nonverbal attending behaviors. Certainly, sustained verbal interaction with others depends to a large extent on whether a person is able to elicit reinforcement, by listening to or exhibiting interest in the statements made by another. Within the present case study, the child's poor attending skills may have discouraged the reinforcing value of conversation, which resulted in the gradual extinction of this social response. By employing positive reinforcement contingencies to appropriate nonverbal attending behavior, the child was able to reestablish ability in making eye contact with persons in his environment. The reestablishment of this response required only six 15-minute training sessions.

These findings support previous research that established nonverbal attending behavior in a language-deficient child (Brooks et al. 1968).

The second component of reestablishing imitative verbal responding, involved the presentation of fifteen objects that were considered valuable or important to the child. During training the subject was presented the object visually and asked to imitate or repeat the trainer's verbal statements about the object. Reinforcement was made contingent upon both appropriate attending and verbalization.

Although this area of training was similar to the procedures used by Lovaas and colleagues (1966), it differed in three distinct ways: (1) emphasis was placed on producing complete verbalizations rather than shaping sounds that approximated words, (2) the fifteen items for training were presented within both auditory and visual modalities, and (3) the subject's parents were utilized as potent sources of positive reinforcement.

During this phase of training the subject reached the response criterion in only five training sessions, suggesting that his motivation remained optimal despite significant reduction of prompting strategies.

Prior to session 18, the child had begun to show a lack of interest in several of the objects being presented during training, while becoming insistent about immediately cashing in tokens for consumables. To prevent response satiation and increase the child's ability to work for delayed reinforcement, a wristwatch was made available for purchase during session 18. This strategy worked well since response criteria were then met during session 19. Simultaneously, appropriate responding for functional language increased from 25 to 40 percent, even though contingent reinforcement had not been established. These findings suggest that even though the child had learned the functional language tasks presented during baseline periods, his motivation for exhibiting this learning (latent learning) was insufficient prior to the introduction of the wristwatch contingency. Generalization required only two trials to criterion when functional language responses were systemically reinforced.

The final component of functional language training involved the contingent reinforcement of verbal responses made to open-ended questions posed by the trainer. The goal of this training was to produce verbal interactions that approximated actual conversation. In many respects this component differed qualitatively from the strategies used by Baer (1968), who was more concerned with the acquisition of functional words and teaching correct grammatical syntax. Since the subject already possessed these skills, interventions were directed at assisting the subject in attending to the trainer's questions and employing appropriate cognitive skills in formulating a coherent and complete verbal response. The expectation was for the subject to move beyond simple imitative speech to constructing relevant sentences.

GENERALIZATION

A systematic approach was used to promote generalization employing strategies developed by Kazdin and Bootzin (1972).

Since a token economy system was used, the same reinforcement contingencies were available throughout all five phases of training. This proved effective in establishing appropriate verbal language and decreased the reliance on immediate primary reinforcement. Response generalization was also promoted by the systematic use of the subject's parents and teachers throughout the training program. This strategy prevented the trainer from becoming the only discriminative stimulus for speech. Future research might profitably be directed at employing other significant social parties such as peers to serve as trainers.

Altering the training setting promoted generalization during the last phase of training. This strategy, coupled with reinforcing appropriate verbal responding in the child's natural environment, proved to be anxiety provoking for the subject. The subject's increased anxiety level certainly helps explain his mild regression in functional language responses during generalization. Although schedules of reinforcement were changed to an FR (4) during this final phase, earlier attempts at fading reinforcement schedules should have been implemented since this abrupt change was distressing for both subject and parents.

In general, the adapted language training program proved to be highly effective in reestablishing verbal language in the 7-year-old child. Both parents and teachers reported a significant increase in verbal interactions with peers and family members outside of training sessions. In addition, progressive and spontaneous verbal interaction was documented at home and school via ongoing observations. His mood was improved and he became less of a behavioral problem at home. The subject's parents also expressed a renewed sense of hope with regard to their role as parents as a result of their participation in the training program.

REFERENCES

American Psychiatric Association. (1987). *Diagnostic and Statistical Manual of Mental Disorders, Third Edition, Revised (DSM-III-R)*. Washington, DC: American Psychiatric Association.

Baer, D. M. (1968). The development of imitation by reinforcing behavior similarity to the model. *Journal of Experimental Analysis of Behavior* 10:405–416.

Baer, D. M., and Guess, D. (1971). Receptive training of adjectival infection in mental retardates. *Journal of Applied Behavior Analysis* 4:129–139.

Barton, E. S. (1972). Operant conditioning of appropriate and inappropriate social speech in the profoundly retarded. *Journal of Mentally Deficient Research* 17:183–191.

——— (1975). The problem of generalization in the operant conditioning of social speech in the severely subnormal. *British Journal of Psychiatry* 127:376–385.

Berrera, R. D., Berrera, D. L., and Sulzer-Azaroff, B. (1980). A simultaneous treatment comparison of three expressive language training programs with a mute autistic child. *Journal of Autism and Developmental Disabilities* 10:21–37.

Blake, P., and Moss, T. (1967). The development of socialization skills in an electively mute child. *Behaviour Research and Therapy* 5:349–356.

Bloom, L. (1970). *Language Development: A Form and Function in Emerging Grammars*. Cambridge, MA: MIT Press.

Borus, J. F. (1973). Establishing imitative speech employing operant techniques in a group setting. *Journal of Speech and Hearing Disorders* 38:533–541.

Bricker, W. A., and Bricker, D. C. (1970). A program of language training for the severely handicapped child. *Exceptional Children* 37:101–111.

Brooks, B. D., Morrow, J. E., and Gray, W. F. (1968). Reduction of autistic gaze aversion by reinforcement of visual attention responses. *Journal of Special Education* 2:307–309.

Evans, I. M. (1971). Theoretical and experimental aspects of the behavior modification approach to autistic children. In *Infan-*

tile Autism: Concepts, Characteristics and Treatment, ed. M. Rutter. Baltimore, MD: Williams & Wilkins.

Fygetakis, L. (1970). Programmed conditioning of linguistic competence. *Behaviour Research and Therapy* 8:153–163.

Garcia, E. (1974). The training and generalization of conversational speech form in non-verbal retardates. *Journal of Applied Behavior Analysis* 7:137–149.

Garcia, E., Baer, D. M., and Firestone, I. (1971). The development of generalized imitation within topographically determined boundaries. *Journal of Applied Behavior Analysis* 4:101–112.

Gray, B. B. (1968). The development of language on a function of programmed conditioning. *Behaviour Research and Therapy* 6:455–460.

Guess, D. A. (1969). A functional analysis of receptive language and productive speech: acquisition of the plural morpheme. *Journal of Applied Behavior Analysis* 2:55–64.

Harris, S. L. (1975). On the importance of being contingent. *Journal of Autism and Childhood Schizophrenia* 4:94–97.

Isaacs, W., Thomas, J., and Goldiamond, I. (1965). Application of operant conditioning to reinstate verbal behavior in mute psychosis. *Journal of Abnormal Psychology* 70:155–164.

Kazdin, A. E., and Bootzin, R. R. (1972). The token economy: an evaluative review. *Journal of Applied Behavior Analysis* 6:343–372.

Koegel, R. L., and Rincover, A. (1974). Treatment of psychotic children in a classroom environment. *Journal of Applied Behavior Analysis* 7:45–60.

Kozloff, M. (1973). *Reaching the Autistic Child: A Parent Training Program*. Champaign, IL: Research Press.

Krolian, E. B. (1988). Speech is silvern, but silence is golden: day hospital treatment of two electively mute children. *Clinical Social Work Journal* 16:4.

Louden, D. M. (1987). Elective mutism: a case study of a disorder of childhood. *Journal of the National Medical Association* 79:10.

Lovaas, O. I., Berberick, J. P., and Perloff, B. F. (1966). Acquisition of speech by schizophrenic children. *Science* 151:705–707.

Marshall, N. R., and Hegrenes, J. (1970). The use of written language as a communication system for an autistic child. *Speech and Hearing* 37:258–261.

Risley, T. R., and Wolf, M. M. (1967). Establishing functional speech in echolalic children. *Behaviour Research and Therapy* 5:73–88.

Sherman, J. A. (1965). Use of reinforcement and imitation to reinstate verbal behavior in mute psychotics. *Journal of Abnormal Psychology* 70:155–164.

PART III

PSYCHODYNAMIC THERAPY

8

ELECTIVE MUTISM: ORIGINS IN STRANGER ANXIETY AND SELECTIVE ATTENTION

Daniel F. Shreeve

THE MUTE CHILD presents a challenge of the first order in therapy, for words are, regardless of the mode of treatment, the tools to secure a working alliance with the patient. Once we have excluded neurological causes, we are left in the room with a child who is able to speak but appears to refuse. Language is such a fundamental part of human relationships that the clinician cannot help but perceive the child's silence as aggressive. In fact, however, only a fraction of these children show a pattern of passive-aggressive behavior or misconduct (Hayden 1980).

In work with the silent child, strong forces act on the psychotherapist to convert from a seeker of meaning to a conqueror of symptoms. The therapist tries to respond more empathically than other adults, who may be presumed to have contributed to the child's disturbance. As Ruzicka and Sackin (1974) described, however, the child's silence inevitably becomes an insult to the therapist's self-esteem. If progress is to be made, the therapist must become fully aware of ongoing countertransferential reactions. A peculiar side effect of the unexplored impact of the child's silence may be a quest for singular explanations of its origin and for specific cures.

From a review of 152 reports on the subject, Hesselman (1983) did not distill a pure or unitary theory for elective mutism; instead we face the awkward problem of having too many good choices! Thus psychoanalytic treatments of the symptom, for example, show that it pertains to the core conflicts of each successive stage of psychosexual development, including oral, anal-rapprochement, and phallic-oedipal phases (Chethik 1973, Radford 1977). Alternatively, mutism can be seen as a family problem, reflecting the use of the child as silent "spokesperson" for the family's distrust of the surrounding culture (Goll 1979). Mutism is surely also a habit, and it has responded favorably to behavioral therapies (Lowenstein 1978), even though certain cases have required the mother's involvement (Croghan and Craven 1982).

Such a menagerie of viewpoints has nonetheless produced the consensus that, whatever the cause of elective mutism, it arises early in the infant's primary phase of attachment. Faulty mother–child interaction, often a pathological symbiosis, is found in numerous case studies (Ambrosino and Alessi 1979, Atoynatan 1986, Wilkins 1985). A predominance of oral fixation is well described by Myquel and Granon (1982): "The mute children draw people with open mouths full of teeth. Games multiply in which animals bite and devour. . . . Open mouths full of teeth, but also closed mouths" (p. 332).

Consistent with this infantile origin, epidemiological studies demonstrate that whereas mutism is often "discovered" at school age, it develops from a prior phase of abnormal timidity (Kolvin and Fundudis 1981). According to Lesser-Katz (1986), a temperamentally shy young child who turns excessively to the mother for reassurance may receive early reinforcement of a fear of strangers. In the context of family pathology, as Myquel and Granon (1982) pointed out, the mother "feels proud and narcissistically reassured by being the only one to whom the child speaks" (p. 333). The stage is thus set for a peculiar intimate exclusiveness of the mother–child dyad that is beyond words. Myquel and Granon described such a union: "They understood one another almost without words, using a nonverbal language of looks and motions" (p. 333).

In the following case report of Clara, I will focus on such an early origin of stillness and on the prelinguistic connotations of silence. I am influenced by the work of Anthony (1977), who initially treated a mute 7-year-old boy by an empathic, silent identification with the child's gestures. Anthony surmised that nonverbal communication is closer to the primary process, and that a major obstacle in therapy is the adult's expectation that words will be spoken. The need to consider primary process is exemplified by Ferenczi's (1923) account of a dream, frequently encountered in psychoanalysis, in which a tiny suckling baby speaks eloquently on profound subjects and expounds grand scientific theories with amazing elocution. Ferenczi believed that, among other meanings, such a dream refers humorously to the analyst's false attribution of logic to the thoughts of the infant.

Insofar as possible, therefore, I entreat the reader to allow multiple and sometimes contrary interpretations of Clara's silence. I contend that an interjection of silence is relatively governed by primary process rules. For example, even in normal adult interactions, the use of the "silent treatment" includes both an implied retaliation for disappointment and the intimation of a longed-for reunion. Zeligs (1961) pointed out that, in psychotherapy, any silence is meaningful as affect-representation, as drive discharge, and as defense. Thus we should be prepared to consider that in work with an electively mute child, the most intense communication may occur in moments of total silence.

CASE REPORT

HISTORY

Clara was almost 4 when she came to our clinic for military dependents. The preschool teacher referred her for evaluation of her "inability" to speak and because the teacher questioned the parents' claim that Clara was in fact precociously verbal at home. Clara, of course, could not comment on this dispute, but stared silently at the interviewer through her thick glasses while clinging to her father. She was small for her age, and her huddled posture made her seem even tinier.

The parents related a history of normal milestones of walking and toilet training, with early speech and self-dressing. Although they were proud of Clara's fine elocution at home, they were fearful that mutism at school could be a harbinger of future mental disorder. Likewise, they worried that Clara's excessive fear of strangers and phobia of insects could be risk factors for adult psychiatric problems. Furthermore, they complained of Clara's oppositionalism, which interfered with the household schedule for meals and bedtime. In the initial sessions, Clara's mother (a registered nurse in the Army) criticized her vigorously, and I had to enforce limits on such criticism when Clara was present.

Further evaluation revealed that each parent secretly hoped that Clara would prove exceptional in school. Clara's tests showed gifted or high-average intelligence scores on all measures, including verbal as well as performance, self-care, and motor coordination. No speech abnormality was discovered, except for extremely low volume (whispering).

Both parents freely admitted long-standing marital conflict, and they eventually confided that the mother was herself in treatment for depression. These problems dated from the beginning of their relationship. The mother, Captain S, reportedly would shout or "throw things" at the climax of a quarrel, whereas Mr. S would avoid confrontations by briefly leaving their home. It was in this setting of perpetual argument that Mr. S often assumed the greater share of parenting duties, including feeding and diapering. Thus Clara's early life was marked both by exposure to loud quarreling and by the mother's partial retreat from parenting. The family's recent history was remarkable for the father's growing success in his career as a professional musician, which had begun to require excursions away from home.

Based on our evaluation, we scheduled Clara for individual psychotherapy and her parents resumed marital therapy, which they had discontinued when the mother was transferred to our area. Thereafter, both parents were punctual throughout the year of treatment, not only in bringing Clara to appointments, but also in their alternating individual sessions with me, as well as in their own marital treatment with another therapist in our clinic.

OBSERVATION AND TREATMENT

Clara and I started work in late summer, just before her preschool began. It was difficult at first to disengage her from her parents for the sessions. She and he father were physically close and often exchanged embraces. In our very first session, immediately after I had persuaded Clara to come from her father's lap to my room, she impressed me with a demonstration of her intellect: At age 4, she could count aloud to 100 and could write all the numbers as well. Without prompting, she next printed her first and last names, each correctly spelled, and on separate pages spelled "mom" and "dad." She seemed pleased with my encouragement and bestowed a fleeting smile on me, but would not respond further that day.

For the next several weeks, Clara lapsed into mutism. My running commentary on the sessions prompted no verbal response from her; when I praised her work, she drew closer but rarely made eye contact. My specific comment on the change in the room to silence merely elicited a frown. Clara recoiled abruptly when I commented that words could be either helpful or scary. I thought that this withdrawal was a familiar reaction to inspection of her symptom, and vowed to abandon direct interrogation about Clara's speech. This dark phase of opening treatment seemed to indicate Clara's rejection not only of my best efforts to wait patiently for her, but also of my most empathic interpretations of her reticence. I actively sought to dismiss words as the goal of treatment, but I nevertheless experienced her mutism as shutting me out, and even as a defeat or devaluation of my efforts.

Captain S, whom I saw alone in these first weeks, continued to express displeasure with her daughter, and she flatly stated that Clara's mutism had intensified since she had started treatment. I felt trapped beneath the weight of impossible demands—I must be gentle and wait quietly for Clara to speak, yet her parents wanted verbal proof of progress.

However well disguised, my desire for speech apparently was known to Clara, who interpreted it as a reproach, which presented another obstacle to her relatedness. As if seeking reassurance that I could not provide, Clara would scan the room furtively. She built play fences around the toy animals and silently made the toy cows kiss. I observed to her that the fence was a protection for the cows and compared her silence to the safety of the fence.

Clara's mother preferred not to accompany her daughter, and in these first months Clara simply stared at me for long intervals, as if oblivious to my interpretations, or even to my presence. She was often absorbed in silent play with the dollhouse. When her father brought her, she was more animated and willing to draw; an early production was that of a smiling man. I asked her about this figure, and she broke the silence by indicating, "My daddy." I commented about the happy face and wondered aloud if Clara wished her father could always be as smiling as he was in the picture. Although she chose not to respond verbally, she began to tidy up the room quite vigorously; I commented about how carefully she took care of messes and suggested that perhaps talking about troubles reminded her of the messes or arguments at home. Because I knew of the parents' quarrels, I pointed out to Clara that she might feel it was her job to "clean up" arguments, but that this task might be too great for her alone.

After about two months of treatment, Clara gave me a warm smile when I arrived in the waiting room. After an initial protest at separating from her mother, Clara settled down silently to drawing the first of many sets of pictures she identified with the labels "Mommy" and "Daddy." These pictures were always the same size, and as identical as she could conceivably make them; she confided in a whisper that they were presents for her parents. I remarked that by giving exactly equal gifts, she must want to "keep everyone happy." This idea seemed to liberate her speech, and she commented that she also had two girlfriends who were spending the night. She made identical pictures for them, too, and I pointed out that she must also want to keep these friends happy by giving them the same gifts. It must be difficult, I added, to balance the worth of presents in this way, especially at times when she might feel like giving more to one person than to another. In a similar context later, I compared this attempt at fairness to her perfectionism as sometimes manifested in how she tidied up the dollhouse, and at other times in how she tried to keep her parents from quarreling.

My interpretations about Clara's wish to "control" her parents would draw a quick frown, but then she would gleefully turn to games such as jack-in-the-box. We eventually achieved an understanding that simple, repetitive play was a relief from unpleasant surprises and from the sudden affective impact of words. Thus supported, Clara visibly relaxed and became more spontaneous in her movements; often, she was even reluctant to leave the room at the end of her session. At this time, her parents were evaluating the therapy, and Clara's father complained to me about her "perfectionistic" traits (I had used this word with Clara but not with the parents).

By the third month, after an initial pause at the start of each therapy session, Clara was interpreting her drawings for me. For example, she commented on the larger mouth of a "mommy" drawing, and she nodded her head when I related this to her mother's anger. Despite Clara's lack of verbal progress at school, I thought the therapy was moving forward. Thus I was not prepared for the next sustained resistance in which Clara completely excluded me from conversation and play for entire sessions. The first incident occurred when I arrived late to take her to the room. She refused to accompany me, so her father joined us; Clara began to speak, but only to her father, and she somehow managed to avoid eye contact with me regardless of how I positioned myself. Clara gazed up at her father from his lap, whispered in his ear, and conducted an independent conversation. I pointed out that she was giving her father a special gift of speech by reserving it for him alone.

About 4 months into Clara's treatment, she and her mother had a stormy argument in the waiting room. When I approached, Clara clung to her mother and refused to separate while her mother chided her loudly and angrily. Captain S repeatedly ordered Clara to go with me, but Clara began to cry, so we elected to conduct the session with her mother in the room. The quarrel began anew in my office, with Clara wailing loudly and her mother vigorously prying Clara's hands away from her arms. Now furious with her daughter, the mother stormed out of the room. Clara then cried nonstop for several minutes, refusing eye contact and, of course, not responding to my words. Only my repeated clarifications about the temporary nature of her mother's fury and its distinction from hatred served to quiet Clara somewhat. I pointed out how much I wished to comfort her, but she seemed to have a wall around her and had become lonely and remote. When Clara's wailing took on a forced, artificial quality, I ended the session; at first sight of her mother, Clara abruptly stopped crying. Mother and daughter left the clinic quietly, at once reconciled and each smiling as if nothing had occurred.

After about six months of treatment, Clara would greet me with a characteristically suspenseful, rather mischievous expression. Her raised eyebrows and tense posture seemed to convey that this moment was special. Yet Clara's eager, almost breathless quality in the waiting room evaporated as soon as we entered my office. A reticent period still marked the start of each session, even though Clara had become more lively and spontaneous in her play. She began to involve me in her activities by telling me how to play with marbles and puppets, or how to draw. Clara often started by dividing some toys exactly in half, then telling me "the rules." I commented on how she measured her portion and mine so evenly, and pointed out that she was also cautious and careful in sharing her words.

As Clara's speech grew more liberated, she also became domineering, a development that was not thwarted by my comments about how controlled I felt, or about how she herself might experience such control outside the room. During this same period, Clara also made our puppets embrace and kiss, and in moments of excitement she complained that the room was too warm. Then, as if to deny this complaint, she would put on her outdoor jacket. Although it was a relief to see Clara smile and become active, I also began to experience her control as isolating and rejecting. I told her that her continual commands made me feel left out.

By early spring (after about seven months of treatment), Clara firmly occupied the role of dictator/teacher. She would give precise, strict instructions on how and when to play games. Jokingly, she would place her hand over the mouth of my puppet to keep it from interrupting, or she would command, "Raise your hand before speaking!" Although Clara insisted that I go through the ritual of raising my hand, she would then nevertheless demand silence and shout, "It's not time now!" Often, Clara wanted to first be the teacher, then to be a pupil with me, both of us working side by side on the assigned "class work." As the teacher, Clara was harsh, but she was also nurturing and protective; as a reward for obedience, she would supply pretend food or perhaps offer special assistance with a drawing.

It was clear that Clara was beginning to internalize an image of her preschool teacher. In fact, her parents reported that Clara had begun to speak in school, softly but at appropriate times. Although her teacher was pleased, her mother now condemned Clara for her extreme need to excel and for demanding too much of the teacher's attention. Both parents cited, as an example, Clara's reluctance to stand in line or await her turn.

After eight months of treatment, Clara seemed dedicated to the art of disregarding my every word, while at the same time engaging me in conversation. If I responded to her productions verbally, she might cover her ears, laughing gaily, or she might simply go on talking as if she had not heard me. It struck me that "not listening" had completely replaced "not speaking." I made this comparison often to Clara, and for brief intervals she would pause as if to consider it.

In desperation, I once asked if she could repeat one of my interpretations and was amazed when she repeated it exactly, word for word!

The next development was Clara's departure from equal sharing. In play, she began to assume the role of "authority," who would greedily appropriate the majority of toys, or the most attractive toys. I commented that by giving in to the teacher, I could earn special approval, but then I would also receive fewer toys. Surprisingly, in separate sessions at this time, the parents were reporting that Clara was finally beginning to share with her peers at school and was also less stubborn at home. Although Captain S was still tentative, she grudgingly admitted progress.

Clara surprised me one day by suddenly stopping a game to reveal a fantasy. With no preamble or warning, she confided that she had been born in an orphanage. Clara explained that her parents had chosen her from among all the other children because she was the prettiest and nicest of all the orphans. Neither parent had heard this story, and I could find no association within the session. About the same time, Clara also startled her parents at home by blurting out, "I'm not to blame for your arguments!" Again, this assertion occurred outside any context we could discern.

At nine months into the therapy, I interpreted one of Clara's silences as being related to her father's unusually harried appearance that day. Clara countered with, "Saying bad things isn't nice!" We were then able to examine the menacing aspect of words and to explore the ideal of being "nice" by not speaking. During this period, Clara began asserting herself in new ways, including—for the first time—making a gift for herself (a drawing of a girl). She continued to create gifts for others; for example, she drew pictures for a girlfriend that she said were designed to "make her happy."

After ten months of treatment, Clara was speaking with good volume and full sentences, and she was also allowing me opportunity to reply. She was, moreover, now quite ready to argue; for example, we debated about whether the best way to secure friends is by being "totally nice." After declaring herself the winner of our discussion, she paused and then abruptly confided again her fantasy of having been "picked out" from an orphanage nursery. During this period, Clara also tried to prevent me from talking to her mother alone by saying, "She doesn't want to see you today." Clara became increasingly reluctant to leave us alone in the room.

By about eleven months of treatment, Clara would organize a cooperative division of activity, instead of neatly assigning us the same tasks or equivalent toys. She became excited by play, and I had to decline her request to join her under my desk in her "hiding place." Frequently, Clara would assign me the role of her favorite friend and would "call" me on the play phone to invite me to "come over and spend the night." Occasionally, she commented rather mechanically, "I love you," on the phone.

During this period, Clara wanted us to alternate in the role of being "it," which she explained to mean "being the teacher." This charade helped us to recognize that teachers, or adults in control, often seemed mysterious, unpredictable, and powerful. For example, Clara, as teacher, rewarded obedience with a "smiley face," but could also suddenly withhold rewards or become harshly scolding. The pupil was presumed to need constant direction, usually issued by the teacher in a brisk, officious manner. Nothing could be undertaken without permission. Furthermore, from Clara's designs for board games, we discovered that the authority figures often broke the rules, despite their apparent rigidity.

Clara now wanted to show her drawings to her mother, but Captain S seemed embarrassed and impatient with this project. When I saw her separately, the mother again complained about Clara's bossiness at home and said, "It gets tiring." I again interpreted Clara's oppositionalism as an aspect of her dependency on her mother. Captain S eventually confided that her impatience was in fact due in part to her husband's absence on business. At this same time, Captain S began to reveal a portion of her actual pride in Clara. When Mr. S returned, the parents began to make further progress in their marital therapy.

After nearly a year of therapy, Clara was no longer inhibited in speech, except for a brief "reminder" of her mutism at the start of each session. She now objected loudly to interpretations she disliked. After I introduced the topic of termination, Clara brought candy for me and would not eat any herself until I accepted it. During her final session, Clara brought a new doll she called "sister." She said she knew all about the ending of treatment, and that it didn't concern her. She devoted much attention to "feeding" and arranging activities for the "sister" doll. She wanted all three of us to sit together at a pretend party and pointed out that the doll should be closest to her, while I should sit a little further away. Using the play phones allowed us to talk about the importance of "the right distance" as well as good-bye feelings.

When summer was over, I reminded Captain S that we had agreed to reevaluate Clara after the start of kindergarten. When the family arrived, I was amazed by Clara, not only by her fast growth to average stature, but especially by the comparative breeziness and self-confidence of her movements. She had brought me a crudely wrapped musical teddy bear, which, judging from the exchange of looks, was also from her mother. Clara wanted all three of us to help put together a puzzle, and loudly objected to her mother's awkward mistakes.

When I met with Captain S alone, she told me that she felt her daughter no longer needed treatment. Clara had acquired friends at school, was handling her schoolwork well, and had excited a special enthusiasm in her new teacher. Both parents were also pleased with the successful conclusion of their marital therapy.

DISCUSSION

Anthony's (1977) analysis of a withdrawn and listless boy demonstrates that elective mutism may be the unspoken complaint of a severe depression; a child may lack almost any energy to reach outward. Clara's bright and mischievous mien required consideration of an alternative etiology because she inspired a lively contest over her gift of speech. Among the various possible causes of her symptomatic mutism, I would suggest origins in the early repertoire of parent–infant interaction. I do not exclude other causes—in particular, Goll's (1979) hypothesis that a parent's general distrust of others can become the model for a child's inhibition with strangers. To the extent that Clara imagined hostility in her mother's remoteness, this perception was split off from the mother–child relationship and projected onto outsiders. Her symptom was a further, elegant solution to the problem of distance, which intensified the state of engagement with her key adult figures while defending against awareness of her dependence on them. By her spells of silence, Clara also retained certain delights of infancy, especially the capacity to summon attention from the caregiver without recourse to speech.

In my work with Clara, I found such infantile meanings first in our puzzling encounters before sessions. What caused her to smile so endearingly, and what was the secret joke that I spoiled with my first words? A possible clue is that Clara knew—like many children—that therapy is a place where one must talk. She anticipated this demand and unconsciously transformed it into a game in which I courted her to accompany me into my office. The game also involved recovering the sight of me, which replaced the memory she held, as well as the reverse: losing sight of her mother while retaining her image.

At actual separation from her mother, though, Clara would panic, and her mother became unsettled by her clinging appeal for reassurance. Clara's sense of rejection would surface in our initial moments alone: At once I became the threatening and fearsome figure, while her mother assumed the image of the comforting caregiver, "absent but present" in opposition to the just-experienced impression of "present but absent." Certainly Clara modeled her silence as an identification with her mother's perceived withholding, and she could project unwanted aspects of the relationship onto me as the adult "stranger."

Clara's sudden stillness in the room resembled the reactions of other electively mute children when they are exposed to strangers, as described by Lesser-Katz (1986, 1988), who suggested an origin for the "freeze-defense" in the reflexive responses of animals to danger.

In children, we see that an abrupt cessation of activity raises the threshold to unwanted aspects of the environment. It is as if the discomforting object can be "wished away" by selective inattention (Hill and Scull 1985). We can compare this reaction to the inhibition of action seen in infants when a parent attempts to alter the direction of play (Bruner 1974); that is, the unwanted stimulus may be merely incongruous rather than dangerous, so that withholding of action reduces the discrepancy between expected and actual parental response. In experimental studies, a parent's neutral rather than smiling expression provokes actual gaze aversion, a defense that minimizes the unpredicted stimulus (Brackbill 1958).

In early childhood, such sensory denial may pertain not only to the environment, but also to the inner world. As Peller (1966) found in his review of Freud (1923), an unconscious memory-trace is first made "external" as a semantic representation before emerging into awareness. Clara, by avoiding language, protected herself not just from the stimuli emanating from a feared object, but also from her own unacceptable affects, including those connected to her mother at the start of sessions. By allowing me to speak, Clara formally distinguished the speaker from the listener and also raised concern to the level of objective scrutiny.

Early in the course of treatment, I thus became identified with the tyranny of the secondary process itself, and therefore with its requirement of goal-directedness and future orientation (see Cottle 1973). I felt alternately like Clara's preschool teacher, who interrupted her daydreams, and as one who rejected the intimation of closeness in her quiet gaze. Without wandering from the subject of Clara's treatment, I would compare the reverie of Clara's long glances to the general predominance of visualization in early childhood experience: Visual memory-pictures give way only gradually to semantic memory and remain heavily invested with affects attached to remembered objects (Lewin 1968). Because of this same phenomenon of subjective recollection, the young child experiences words not purely as instrumental but as the perception of the symbolized object that actually intrudes into awareness (Greenson 1950). Words not only interrupt fantasy; they also force attention toward an externally chosen point.

Against the imposition of these demands of language, Clara maintained both strict limits for her participation and an autocratic rule over all of our interactions in therapy. A long struggle for control preceded her tolerance for interpretations, or even for the mutuality of conversation. I would argue that affinity for language pertains to the control struggles of rapprochement in a way parallel to the development of other faculties, including motor skills: Growth in capacities paradoxically brings acquaintance with realistic limitations. Reliance on speech involves the essential discovery that the parent can no longer be summoned magically through hallucinations as in infancy, but only by verbal efforts and subject to variable delays. The toddler finds compensation for this loss in a reasonable expectancy of the mother's return, an important precedent for the growth of time orientation and the emergence of secondary process (Hartocollis 1974). Words then become useful in defining separate experiences with the parent, interfering with a singular image based on wishes. Such achievements in object relations, of course, normally precede advanced verbal skills.

To consider what deficits could have affected Clara's rejection of speech, we may note first those steps in early life toward mutuality that require the parent's empathic attention—in particular, a sharing of focus of attention and the parent's facilitation of the child's gestures or intentions (Stern 1985). A newfound intersubjectivity and a sense of personal agency, predicated on the parent's attunement to need, serve to restore calm in the setting of a growing awareness of individuation. The bipolar, joint actions of mother–infant play provide a model for the essential language dichotomies of subject versus object, initiator versus recipient of action, and cause versus effect (Bruner 1974, Inhelder 1971). Even the infant's awareness of inner affective states depends on observing countless reactions of the parent. Indeed, this synchrony or reciprocal interaction is such a constant feature of parenthood that it can be considered inborn and driven by a biological preparedness (Emde 1989).

Yet multiple forms of misattunement may affect the parent–infant relationship, thus introducing irregularity into the approach of infant to parent (Lichtenberg 1989). Whereas ideally a mother is in a perpetual state of readiness to perceive and empower the child's actions, such perfection is rarely achieved. Here we find a premise for the control struggle of rapprochement in the variable ability to influence the more powerful adult figures. To the extent that the toddler feels helpless and alone, the parent's receptiveness may be fantasized as a susceptibility to control.

It is to this stage, at the time of the toddler's first words, that I believe Clara returned to rework essential advances in object relations. By the use of her silence, Clara held the eyes of key adult figures, a primitive sharing of the suspense in waiting which was, of course, far from mutual in its enjoyment. This creative use of silence by Clara may be compared to the general ethological observation that an interpolated pause may enhance the significance of proximate message units (R. Capranica, personal communication, 1990). Here again we find a parallel in the life of infants, for our soliciting of the infant's responses normally involves silent pauses that allow for the infant's reciprocal action. In unconscious adjustment to communication with an infant, the adult commonly exaggerates the melody of speech while interspersing poignant pauses, so that silence becomes a tool of affective engagement (P. Kuhl, personal communication, 1990).

I believe that a similar constructive use of silence was possible for Clara because her mother did not exhibit misattunement in the form of actual indifference. Rather, we may surmise that Captain S was outspoken in her criticism of Clara because she was more profoundly attached to her young daughter than she could initially profess. Clara was not oblivious to the latent possibilities of greater relationship and unconsciously played on this restriction in her willful contests over speech. Clara's mother modeled a steady progress in her capacity for relationship and eventually achieved a relatively open display of affection. This reorientation enabled Clara to relinquish a distorted image of silence as the symbol of attachment. In time, Clara gave up her reminiscence of an imaginary parent, one whose voice conveyed only the preverbal signs of emotion, and who made no demand for reply.

ACKNOWLEDGMENTS

I am grateful to Jerron Adams, M.A., for her skillful and successful collateral therapy with the parents. Todd Larsen, Ph.D., and Kristine Terry, Ph.D., contributed valuable ideas and suggestions during the writing. For translations from the French, I thank Mrs. Mauricette Fairley.

REFERENCES

Ambrosino, S. V., and Alessi, M. (1979). Elective mutism: fixation and the double bind. *American Journal of Psychoanalysis* 39:251–256.

Anthony, E. J. (1977). Nonverbal and verbal systems of communication: a study in complementarity. *Psychoanalytic Study of the Child* 32:307–325. New Haven, CT: Yale University Press.

Atoynatan, T. H. (1986). Elective mutism: involvement of the mother in the treatment of the child. *Child Psychiatry and Human Development* 17:15–27.

Brackbill, Y. (1958). Extinction of the smiling response in infants as a function of the reinforcement schedule. *Child Development* 29:115–124.

Bruner, J. S. (1974). The ontogenesis of speech acts. *Journal of Child Language* 2:1–19.

Chethik, M. (1973). Amy: the intensive treatment of an elective mute. *Journal of the American Academy of Child Psychiatry* 12:482–498.

Cottle, T. J. (1973). Memories of half a life ago. *Journal of Youth and Adolescence* 2:201–212.

Croghan, L. M., and Craven, R. (1982). Elective mutism: learning from the analysis of a successful case history. *Journal of Pediatric Psychology* 7:85–93.

Emde, R. N. (1989). The infant's relationship experience: developmental and affective aspects. In *Relationship Disturbances in Early Childhood: a Developmental Approach*, ed. A. J. Sameroff and R. N. Emde, pp. 33–51. New York: Basic Books.

Ferenczi, S. (1923). The dream of the "clever baby." In *Further Contributions to the Theory and Technique of Psycho-Analysis*, pp. 349–350. London: Hogarth, 1950.

Freud, S. (1923). The ego and the id. *Standard Edition* 19:1–66.

Goll, K. (1979). Role structure and subculture in families of elective mutists. *Family Process* 18:55–68.

Greenson, R. R. (1950). The mother tongue and the mother. *International Journal of Psycho-Analysis* 31:18–23.

Hartocollis, P. (1974). Origins of time: a reconstruction of the ontogenetic development of the sense of time based on object-relations theory. *Psychoanalytic Quarterly* 43:243–261.

Hayden, T. L. (1980). Classification of elective mutism. *Journal of the American Academy of Child Psychiatry* 19:118–133.

Hesselman, S. (1983). Elective mutism in children 1877–1981. *Acta Paedopsychiatrica* 49:297–310.

Hill, L., and Scull, J. (1985). Elective mutism associated with selective in activity. *Journal of Communication Disorders* 18:161–167.

Inhelder, B. (1971). The sensory-motor origins of knowledge. In *The Development of Self-Regulatory Mechanisms*, ed. D. N. Walcher and D. L. Peters, pp. 141–155. New York: Academic Press.

Kolvin, I., and Fundudis, T. (1981). Elective mute children: psychological development and background factors. *Journal of Child Psychology and Psychiatry and Allied Disciplines* 22:219–232.

Lesser-Katz, M. (1986). Stranger reaction and elective mutism in young children. *American Journal of Orthopsychiatry* 56:458–469.

——— (1988). The treatment of elective mutism as stranger reaction. *Psychotherapy* 25:305–313.

Lewin, B. D. (1968). *The Image and the Past*. New York: International Universities Press.

Lichtenberg, J. D. (1989). *Psychoanalysis and Motivation*. Hillsdale, NJ: Analytic Press.

Lowenstein, L. F. (1978). A summary of research on elective mutism. *Acta Paedopsychiatrica* 44:17–22.

Myquel, M., and Granon, M. (1982). Le mutisme électif extrafamilial chez l'enfant: A propos de quatorze observations [Extrafamilial elective mutism in children, in connection with 14 observations]. *Neuropsychiatrie de l'Enfance* 30:329–339.

Peller, L. E. (1966). Freud's contribution to language theory. *Psychoanalytic Study of the Child* 21:448–467. New York: International Universities Press.

Radford, P. (1977). A psychoanalytically-based therapy as the treatment of choice for a six-year-old elective mute. *Journal of Child Psychotherapy* 4:49–65.

Ruzicka, B. B., and Sackin, H. D. (1974). Elective mutism: the impact of the patient's silent detachment upon the therapist. *Journal of the American Academy of Child Psychiatry* 13:551–561.

Stern, D. N. (1985). *The Interpersonal World of the Infant: A View from Psychoanalysis and Developmental Psychology*. New York: Basic Books.

Wilkins, R. (1985). A comparison of elective mutism and emotional disorders in children. *British Journal of Psychiatry* 146:198–203.

Zeligs, M. A. (1961). The psychology of silence: its role in transference, countertransference and the psychoanalytic process. *Journal of the American Psychoanalytic Association* 9:7–43.

9

ELECTIVELY MUTE CHILDREN: A THERAPEUTIC APPROACH

Otto Weininger

I WILL BEGIN with a brief overview of the literature on elective mutism in children and then discuss my own theoretical position and clinical experience, focusing on two specific cases.

Hesselman (1983) provides us with a concise working definition: it is a condition whereby children who are not psychotic and who can communicate verbally, talk only to certain people, usually significant others in their lives.

With slight variations, electively mute children are typically described in the literature as being especially close to their mothers. Although they are verbal with the immediate family, they refuse to speak to strangers who come to the house. They are usually brought for treatment when they begin school since they will not speak to teachers or other children. Despite their apparent inhibition with strangers, they can be quite demanding and stubborn at home, indicating that although they seem passive, they in fact actively hold themselves back from speaking.

Elective mutism generally becomes apparent when children are

around 3 to 6 years of age, although cases have been reported beginning in and lasting into adolescence (Kaplan and Escoll 1973).
Some studies suggest a higher incidence in girls, while others con-
clude a fairly equal split between the sexes.

The families of these children are frequently "closed" to the outside world. Marital discord is common. In the literature the mothers are often described as enmeshed with the child while the fathers
are referred to as being uninvolved and passive (Meyers 1984).

As a symptom, elective mutism appears to be rare, although
some authors writing in the psychological literature suspect there are
many undetected cases. Some studies (e.g., Bradley and Sloman 1975)
report that a high proportion of elective mutes come from immigrant
families, with the proportion of cases reported highest in the kindergarten population, perhaps indicating family and separation problems experienced by these children.

VARIETIES OF INTERPRETATION

Interpretations of elective mutism differ. Many authors view the
symptom as passive-aggressive behavior. Social learning theorists
(Blotcky and Looney 1980) see it as an acquired way of reducing fear
and anxiety, avoiding unpleasantness, and obtaining privileges and
attention. (Their teachers spend considerable time with these children encouraging them to speak.) Learning theorists point to the
modeling of such behavior on a "quiet" parent, frequently the father.

Psychodynamic writers (Anthony 1977) emphasize its controlling, withholding aspects. Some view it as a denial of oral aggression, others as a fixation of, or regression to, the anal libido stage.

Systems theorists point to the family dynamics: a closed family
system, an enmeshed mother–child relationship, and an emotionally
unavailable father. Since mothers in recently immigrated families are
more vulnerable to feelings of isolation due to language and cultural
barriers, these characteristics may be exaggerated in such families.

The most effective treatment for elective mutism appears to be individual psychotherapy with a focus on empathetic understanding of the child. Collaborative work with the family and the school is also necessary. Behavioral approaches are not as appropriate because they interfere with the child's defenses in a coercive way and make demands on a child prior to his or her capacities to integrate the demand expectation. Rewarding a child because he or she makes an utterance does not mean that the child is ready to speak. Withdrawing further rewards until speech is again present, arouses feelings of inadequacy and adds to the burden of maintaining the mutism. A case report by Crema and Kerr (1978) describes how a child receiving such treatment became even more resistant to speaking. Inpatient treatment, that is, removal from the home, is also of questionable value because of problems of separation.

Treatment of individual cases of elective mutism has been reported by psychoanalytically oriented therapists. The main focus of this approach is to understand the meaning of the child's silence rather than to elicit speech. Anthony (1977), in a very sensitive account of his work with a 7-year-old mute boy, describes how the child communicated with him nonverbally for four months before feeling secure enough to speak. The child's relationship with the analyst enabled him to communicate his feelings through play, with the analyst at times acting as the boy's voice.

CLINICAL EXPERIENCE AND THEORETICAL APPROACH

In my own practice I have seen elective mutism in children 3 to 6 years of age and the majority have been girls. These children seemed to suffer a crisis related to separation from the family when they started school, whether day-care, nursery, preschool, or regular public school, which reflected an inner experience of suspicion toward the outside world. These children began to experience anxiety in trying to maintain themselves in a new situation. They often felt that they were not going to be able to "hold" themselves together. These children were not psychotic. The problem seemed to be an effort to maintain ego-control over aggressive feelings. The conflict was between an inability to express dependency and a basic desire for closeness. So the silence functioned in two ways to maintain a form of ego integrity: If these children did not talk, they did not risk shouting, or saying something nasty. At the same time, if they did not talk, the teacher paid more attention to them and demonstrated more concern. Thus, both aggressive and dependency needs were satisfied by not talking.

As mentioned, this situational crisis was often occasioned by beginning school. Ego functioning was poor and the mother was required to be an auxiliary ego control. However, their mothers were not in the class with these children. Their desire for control related to the fear of expressing sadistic feelings and to projective identification. Projective identification serves as a bridge between the inner world of the child and the external relationships, essentially, a bridge between internal and external reality. In elective mutism, projective identification serves as a method of communicating with the parent.

Projective identification is the projection of certain parts of the ego into the parent, in this case mother, and then forcefully controlling, and simultaneously identifying with her. This form of communication serves to make the child become aware of her or his projection because of the dangers of retaliation from the mother, thereby creating a form of interpersonal relationship (Crisp 1986). A necessary splitting of good and bad aspects takes place within the thinking of the child, and the bad feelings and impulses are projected into the mother. The mother now contains those bad bits, which were dangerous for the child to hold onto, and protects the child from the hostility that is projected into her. By talking only to the mother, the child controls her: the child tells her what to do, and, often, how to do things. Having gained such circular satisfaction, the child is able to maintain silence with others, and is sustained in turn by the intensified concern generally expressed by the mother and/or parents as well as by others outside the family.

The mother of such a child may be passive in relating to the father, and she is often isolated from others. She may unconsciously present the child with the opportunity of projecting hostility into her, while at the same time offering solace to the child because the child talks only with her. The child is angry and cannot seem to do anything about his or her anger and feels helplessly lonely. By identifying with a mother who has similar unconscious feelings about others, the child controls his or her feelings. The child now has the illusion of having no "bad feelings," and can "function" in school, except for talking and friendship.

Projection and the splitting of bad and good are normal processes of psychic growth, but the excessive splitting and projective identification of the electively mute child are the result of persecutory anxiety. For such a child to express anger is to suffer imagined fearful retaliation and therefore persecution. An immature ego lessens the child's opportunity to test reality and see this reality as "friendly" or accepting, and so the mutism continues. At home the child is negative, argumentative, stubborn, and difficult to manage, even with his or her mother. But, because all these qualities are now contained within the mother, they are shown mainly at home and with her. The child has to control the mother in order to control the impulses in him or herself.

In the children I have worked with, the following ego functions were usually immature or ineffective: the ability to deal with situations, to express their needs, to be angry appropriately, to tell another person what they want to do, or ask anything of that person.

The parents usually describe their children as very demanding at home, needing to have things done right away, and always insisting that their mother do things with them. The father, in the cases I saw, is usually uninvolved and, as the literature notes, is usually not a very verbal person. Understandably, teachers, usually primary-grade teachers, tend to to be very concerned and protective of these children. The children seem to ask the teacher for the kind of protection that mothers usually provide. None of the families I have worked with were immigrants.

EVA

When I began to work with Eva, she had been mute for seven months. An only child, she had stopped talking at about 5 years of age when she entered school. Pretty and quiet, she seemed to attract people to her. Though she never spoke, she smiled, and she seemed to give the feeling that she did not want to bother anyone. Occasionally she was heard to say something to an older girl in the playground, but she rarely spoke to any other children. This older girl seemed to be more of a mother than a friend and as such could always "take care" of Eva.

I worked with this little girl in play psychotherapy for about four months. At first, her play was totally nonverbal. The toys I chose were a family of doll toys and a toileting set including a little toilet, a bathtub and a sink, small dollhouse furniture, and paper, pencil, and crayons. Her play theme was primarily toileting the girl and the mother together, and my interpretations were directed toward the anal sadistic activity usually focused on the little girl doll.

Often in the early psychotherapy sessions the scene involved a family, composed of a boy, a girl, a mother, and a father. Mother always took the little girl to the toilet and made her sit on and look into the toilet. The girl doll and mother doll would then look in the toilet together. I said, "I think that they need to see the poo because sometimes poo is bad and makes people very angry," and she looked at me but did not say anything. She then took the pencil and started scratching furiously on the paper. I said, "I think that you are very angry but it's hard for you to tell me how angry you are because you don't like me talking about the poo. You want the mommy to see the poo and not be hurt." She continued to scratch furiously. This play continued in the following sessions.

After four weeks of twice a week sessions, Eva spoke, saying, "The poo stays in the toilet." And I said, "Yes, the poo stays in the toilet." This exchange, essentially, confirmed that the dangerous "poo" would not escape and destroy her or her mother. I felt that it was very important not to push this child to talk as this might re-

duce her ego defenses. I was trying to create a safe relationship, to
help allay her anxieties through interpretation and in this way to
open the way for any possible dialogue with her. Eva later added,
"Nobody is going to take the poo out." She said, "The poo doesn't
jump out by itself." I said, "No, poo doesn't jump out by itself." She
said, "It splashes." I said, "Well I think sometimes when you poo it
does make a splash." And she said, "The splash could really hurt
you." I said, "Why?" No answer. I said, "Well, sometimes people think
that poo is very bad. Sometimes they think that when it gets on
you, that it could hurt you." She said, "Yes." What I was relating
was that she perceived feces as a destructive, harmful, hurtful agent
and whenever she pooed she had to have Mommy come to see that
the poo was contained in the toilet bowl and that the girl and mother
were all right. The mother became the container for the bad impulses
and had to say that the girl was a good girl and the poo would go
away and not hurt the mother as well.

Eva's fantasy play confirmed the good and bad split, and the
projection of the bad into mother and identification with her were
also clarified. Interestingly, when I met with the family, we talked
about her toilet training and the difficulties that they had and how
she was so afraid of defecating in her pants. I think that the child
was very concerned, not that she was going to defecate when she
was in school, but that the fantasized unconscious "badness" that
she felt was in her was going to come out when she spoke while away
from mother. In other words, the sadistic fantasy associated with
defecation was symbolically replaced as not speaking.

After the four months that we worked together, Eva continued talking and seemed to have no further problems that I know
of. (I had told the mother and father that they were free to call and
we could discuss any problems on the phone.) The teacher found
her a very bright and talkative child in class.

I saw this child's problem not simply as an inability to separate
from mother, as we might find in school-phobia difficulty, but rather
as a fear that leaving mother and being in a classroom might not
enable her to have control over her projections. The expression of

aggression was symbolized in her fantasies about her feces. Theoretically, I view this child's problem as an early anal sadistic fantasy and that is why I chose the family and toileting scene for the play psychotherapy. This doesn't necessarily mean that the anal period was difficult or toilet training was hard. What is important is the fantasy that the child has in terms of his or her own goodness and sense of ego integration in relationship to the mother and father.

In terms of this family's dynamics, the mother was the dominant person while the father was relatively passive. She made all domestic decisions, including planning outings, entertaining, and buying new things for the house. The father went along with her. He was frequently away from the house; he worked, but rarely talked about his job at home. The mother did not know very much about his work, partly because he did not want to talk about it. She was in charge at home and father outside of the home and there was little connection, or discussion, between them.

The primary focus of the family dynamics was the daughter's identification with the mother. The mother's modus operandi was, if things were done well at home, one did not worry too much about outside of the home. Similarly, the daughter attempted to make sure that everything in the home was "good, done well and nicely." The daughter imagined that to do something outside of the home would be aggressive. However, she was not able to express this aggression as a result of persecutory anxiety. She thought her parents would perceive her as not being the nice, kind, loving little daughter that she fantasized she must be. She would lose them and the containment they provided.

Individual play psychotherapy was chosen because the child's presenting problem was not of long standing and she did have sufficient ego strength to undergo treatment. In addition, family therapy was rejected by the parents as they did not see themselves as having any problems. To insist upon this type of therapy may have resulted in losing the child as well as the family. Since the parents saw their daughter as having a serious problem they agreed to meet from time to time.

As you work with a child, you inevitably create changes in the parents. In this case, the mother was freed of her child's projections and perhaps of some of her own inhibitions. As the daughter talked more outside, the mother also started doing more outside, as if following her daughter's lead. This made it even easier for the daughter. The father and the mother also seemed to be communicating more, as evident in the last interview, when they were both making decisions regarding their family trip. The child's growth, as he or she develops psychologically, demands that the family system change—or, unfortunately, sometimes break apart. In this case positive changes took place in the family.

SUE

In Sue's case, elective mutism had been present for about three years. Sue was a 6-year-old girl with two older brothers. Her only problem was described as refusing to speak in school. In grade 1 she spoke to only two or three children, but never in class or in school. At home she talked to some children, but not to others; the teachers described her as a "model" student showing no problems except for mutism. She had always been reluctant to talk to anyone outside of the immediate family. Her mother described her as someone who disliked "tidying up and speaking" or interacting with nonfamily members. She had many interests—arts and crafts, skiing, skating, ballet, gymnastics—and apparently was good at everything.

Her medical history was uneventful. She did have her tonsils and adenoids operated on because of frequent ear infections, but there were no complications. No unusual developmental problems were reported. Toilet training was not a problem and she was toilet-trained at 2½ years. She said her first words at about 12 months: "light," and "mommy" and "daddy." She was talking in sentences by 2 to 2½ years, but when she went into nursery school at 3, she did not talk outside of her home.

At home Sue talked a lot; she had to compete with two brothers who were also talkers and she often fought with them. Sue was extremely independent, wanting to do everything for herself. At times however, she acted as though she were helpless. For example, Sue's father indicated she would ask him very politely to do things for her that she did not seem to be able to do by herself. Both parents let Sue have her way and seemed to be quite careful about not upsetting her. Her father described their interaction as sometimes like "walking on eggs." She was touchy and took things very personally, saying her "parents don't like me." Often, Sue thought her mother was angry with her and even when her mother was just reading, Sue would ask her, "Why are you angry with me?"

In our first session, Sue seemed very hesitant, standing at the door speculating whether to come in or to go with her mother. I said "sometimes it's hard to leave Mommy and come into a room with someone you've only met once." Sue then came in, stood in the middle of the room, and stared at the floor for about 5 minutes. Then I showed her the play materials I had brought—a dollhouse with furniture, a number of animals, paper, glue, scissors, tape, string, and a family of dolls. The family of dolls had a father, two mothers (one who was neatly dressed and the other sloppily clothed), two boy dolls, a girl doll, and a baby doll.

Sue first lined all the crayons up neatly and when I asked her if she wanted to make a picture, she nodded her head yes and did three drawings. In one she drew different-colored lines, a girl with colors around her head, a small monkey-shaped creature, a flower and a sun; she then covered the picture with rain marks. I suggested that the girl was trying to keep everything in her head, not letting anything out, and not letting anything in. Sue nodded her head yes. I suggested that the monkey-like creature was a small boy and since he had what seemed to be a middle leg, I indicated that this was a boy's penis, that this was his way of peeing. Sue looked at me, smiled, and then drew rain all over the painting. I suggested that Sue was sometimes afraid that pee would destroy everything and that her brothers could pee on things and that she couldn't. Then Sue nodded yes. I suggested that all the colored lines around her head were to keep the pee out and protect her. She nodded yes and at this time went to the dollhouse and began to organize all the furniture. She placed all the furniture in various rooms and during this entire time neither frowned nor smiled, but kept a deadpan face. When the session was over she left without smiling, and walked down the hall with her mother without talking.

In our next session, Sue came into the room with a blank look, an expressionless face while she hesitated to leave her mother. She simply looked at her and walked through the door. Sue stood looking at the floor and when I suggested that we could play with the materials, she dropped to her knees, and began to play with the house, organizing the furniture the same way as the last session. Then she put the mother wearing the torn dress and the father in bed together. The boys were in one bed and the girl in the crib. I said to Sue that she wanted to be the baby and get all the good stuff from Mommy, but the mommy was a torn mommy, who was trying to get some good stuff from the daddy so that she could give it to the baby. Sue nodded yes, took the girl from the crib and put her into bed with the parents, then threw the father doll across the room, leaving the torn-dressed mother with the girl together. I interpreted this to Sue that she was now going to try and get the good stuff from this mommy, but this mommy didn't seem to be the good mommy. Sue took the doll with the torn dress and heaved her across the room and left the girl in the parents' bed.

I suggested to Sue that she was now alone in bed, wondering where she was going to get the stuff that she needed and that maybe she was afraid that the parents would be angry with her. At this point she took all the animals and began to sort them. She hid the ferocious animals, such as the tiger, lion, and alligator, under boxes, while she placed the domestic animals, such as the sheep, cows, horses, goats, and pigs, beside the house. I said that she wanted to make sure that the animals that could hurt were hidden, and that sometimes she would like to scratch and eat up Mommy and Daddy, but was afraid of her feelings. While she could think them, it was hard to say them. Sue brought out the alligator and began to attack the mother in the untorn dress with it, poking the tail of the alligator into the genitals of the mother. She then had it bite the anus and the breasts of the mother and began to make what could only be described as gleeful cackling noises. She brought mother and father together and began banging them on each other and I indicated that the mother would get the good penis from the father and be able to give it to Sue. She used sounds, mainly aggressive, gutteral ones, and at times she laughed aloud. There was much movement with a lot of throwing of animals and people about.

The next session was almost a repetition of the previous session, except that she said "no" and made lots of sounds. She responded when I interpreted her oral sadistic behavior by throwing the animals and people about. While she seemed very angry, she also smiled a lot.

In our next session the parents sent a note saying that Sue was "very reluctant and anxious about coming to the past sessions and complained that she had stomachaches." But at this session she "was happy and very relaxed," and in the note the parents wrote that she said, "He's not a doctor, he's a player." This session was much noisier, very aggressive, a lot of throwing of animals, sorting them, hiding them. After I interpreted her sadistic acts toward the father doll, she made a penis out of plasticene for father, mother, brother dolls, but not for the girl doll. She pushed the penises into the small toilet in the dollhouse, making gurgling, cackling sounds. Then she became very quiet and wanted me to clean up the room. As I cleaned, she made a drawing which I interpreted as an attempt at reparation so that I would not be angry or hurtful to her. The drawing had a lot of lines, with a very strong border which I interpreted as her wish to have her hostile and sadistic impulses contained. She was afraid of her feelings of wanting to destroy and control and also to get a penis from the mother.

After two weeks of psychotherapy, Sue arrived for the session smiling. Yet, as she was sorting the animals, I felt that she was very sad and I said so. She nodded her head, finished sorting the animals into the aggressive and domestic animals, fixed the house up, and made some very "covered over" drawings in which she put lines on top of lines to obliterate what she had drawn. Sue seemed very uncomfortable and I asked her if she had a tummy ache. She nodded her head yes, and I asked if she wanted to do anything about it. I interpreted her tummy ache and her sadness as fear that her anger would make her mommy and daddy angry with her and that too much of her anger had come out. She was afraid that she could not hold onto it. She continued drawing one line on top of another indicating again her attempt to cover over and maybe even bury her feelings. At about this point tears were streaming down her face and I told her that her feelings were not going to hurt her mommy and daddy, and it was safe to express them in the room, that I would not get angry with her, nor would I throw her away like she wanted to throw the dolls away. Sue looked at me, took the scissors and began to cut the drawing into small pieces as if she was trying to cut her sadism into small bits so it would be less dangerous.

In the next few sessions Sue produced a lot of drawings, which included "covering over" and "surrounding" of objects or colors. I interpreted her fear that her feelings might get "loose" and hurt her mommy, and pointed out her attempt to protect her insides from being hurt as well as her feelings from going out.

In our next session I pointed out to Sue how unhappy she was last time and that her tummy ache was part of her unhappiness and that she was a very sad little girl because she was afraid of her strong feelings. Sue nodded yes. She indicated that she didn't want to play with the house, but wanted to draw pictures. Again, she drew completely closed objects. Some of them had spikes on them as if to protect or/and keep people away. In her final drawing of the session she drew a very closed-in house, although with a door and door handle. Then on either side of the house she drew heart-like objects. On one side the hearts were made into pillar-like objects, while on the other they were scattered, although contained within a blue field. I suggested that maybe she was drawing hearts for the house and that maybe the house would feel better and the hearts would enter the house. At one side of the house there were daddy hearts, on the other, mommy hearts; the house seemed to be "Sue House" and that maybe the daddy and the mommy hearts were going to be kind and loving to the Sue House and give the Sue House the hearts that she needed. Sue smiled in response to this and I said, "I think that you are happier when the mommy and daddy hearts feel like they are inside you and not hurting you." Again, she smiled and nodded her head and our session ended. She walked toward her father who had brought her and was waiting for her. He made no comment to her or myself nor did he show any sign of feeling.

During the next few sessions Sue looked very sad. She indicated to me that she did not want to play with any of the materials, but only to draw and that she also did not want me to talk. She would not allow me to interpret the drawings which shared an enclosed controlled, rigid style so that no movement of either the girl or the cat that she drew was possible. In one she drew a cemetery with gravestone markers and I said that this picture told me she did not want to let her feelings live, that she was afraid that they would get her into trouble and hurt her mommy and daddy. Following this she made a series of numbers. These again indicated control and I interpreted her anxiety about being with me and how her feelings became very strong when we played and this frightened her. Tears streamed down her face and she put her hand to her mouth showing me she did not want me to talk. She continued to make rigid drawings, all contained by lines drawn around the figures and objects so that there was no possibility that any feelings might leak out.

In our next session Sue appeared very pleasant, smiled at me, and immediately began her enclosed drawings. She then cut out part of her drawing so that it formed a kind of door. She quickly made a figure that looked like a child and put it behind the door so that she could open the door and see this figure. I said that it looked like the little girl wanted to come out through the door and that maybe she was not as frightened of her feelings now and could begin to show them more and not be worried that I would be angry at her for showing them. Sue threw the animals around the room and then gathered them, lined them up, hid some, had animals chewing on each other, and lined up the crayons, followed by throwing them about the room. She was very aggressive, messy, destructive; she smiled and made grunting noises. Periodically Sue looked at her construction, opening the door and looking at the little girl. I interpreted this as the little girl coming out of the room in which she had been locked and not being afraid, feeling sometimes angry and sometimes sad, but also sometimes happy. Sue nodded and this time she folded her construction and when I asked whether she was going to give it to her mother, Sue smiled and nodded yes.

At the end of this session I learned from my secretary that Sue's mother had said that Sue was now speaking to her teacher in a "loud whisper." Speech is an early sublimation and when a high-order ego defense mechanism does not develop, hostility that would be directed toward the mother for fantasized withholding of good objects would then be expressed by projection, followed by fear of retaliation. At first, Sue's behavior in the playroom seemed to be an attack upon the fantasized mother. When the mother withheld, Sue attacked the father. Both were ungiving, and she threw them to the other end of the room. When she collected them, she had them perform sexual intercourse, but this time the intercourse was with the good mother and again Sue attempted to gain the penis that she fantasized the mother had given to the father. The envy appeared so overwhelming that Sue could do little except to bring out the destructive animal, the alligator, and chew her mother to pieces, but then, the fantasized retaliation was too great and Sue hid the animals in boxes so that they were no longer visible to her. Yet it was apparent that even hiding the animals was not sufficient. The fantasy was too strong and her reaction was sadness accompanied by a sick stomach.

In the latter instance I think that Sue felt that her own insides were being damaged and that she was punished for having tried to make sadistic attacks upon the mother. Her own destructive impulses resulted in feared retaliation. When the penises were put into the toilet and as the bits of plasticene were squashed into the toilet bowl, Sue had such difficulties with play that she gradually stopped playing with the house furniture and the animals, did not want to see them anymore, and insisted that they be put away. She now concentrated on her drawings which were closed in, covered over; aggressive drawings, yet with a feeling of being contained, indicating that her aggressive fantasies were no longer going to attack. She explored the world of her drawings and showed her aggressiveness in coloring and scribbling.

Gradually, Sue was able to formulate her drawings so that they could become reparation to her mother. As this happened, she began to vocalize farting sounds—loud, long, and full of saliva. She was able to throw crayons about the room, hurtling the objects as an expression of aggression and in that way, perhaps ridding herself of some of the hostility, while at the same time expressing it directly. It appeared that through this aggressive expression, coupled with the reparative nature of her drawings, Sue was able to sublimate her feelings and to gradually use words in the classroom. Her drawings also became aggressive, in that she used crayons as jabbing instruments, almost as though they had now become the hostile penis. After making the drawings she would indicate that she was going to take them home, and when I asked her if she was going to give them to her mother, to make her mother feel good, Sue nodded yes. She would then throw the crayons about the room as if she was throwing these hostile penises away and look at me with a smile on her face. I interpreted this to mean that she felt more like a girl and like her mommy to which she nodded and smiled broadly.

Her projective identification would appear to be her way of formulating an interpersonal relationship with others in her external world. This young girl's way of defending herself against the possibility of retaliation for her hostility was to project her aggression onto her mother. The anxiety that this projection aroused was diminished by her demands upon the mother that she do things "perfectly" and were issued in loud aggressive verbal terms. She was able to express her sadism by direct attacks on her brothers, attacks that were meant to rob them of their penises. She tried to give these organs back to mother in an attempt to control her own sadistic impulses toward her mother, which were dangerous because she feared retaliation. The ego, in an attempt to maintain itself, projected its sadism into mother to damage the mother and at the same time protect itself.

This young girl attempted to maintain control by sorting the wild and domestic animals, and then periodically bringing out some of the fierce ones and attacking the human figures, in particular the mother. At about this point in her play, she began to throw the animals and the people about the room and laughing aloud. This was followed by a very quiet period in the same session and she made drawings that she later took home to her mother as, I think, a form of reparation and the expression of the development of creativity. The mother as a good object could save her daughter and as a bad object could destroy her daughter. The child's attempts to control her own feelings so that they did not provoke the bad feelings in her mother was split off but was demonstrated by the child's periodic sadistic use of the alligator to eat at the bum and breasts of the mother wearing the torn dress, which I called the "bad mother." When she could control, or felt that she could control the bad mother, she threw the mother doll away and took the good mother doll and put her with the father, and then put her with the daughter. Perhaps in fantasy this demonstrated intercourse and mutual reparation and the mother was able to provide some of this to the daughter. This was never done aggressively, but lovingly and kindly. By strengthening the identification with the good mother, the daughter saw the mother as containing good parts of herself and not being a separate individual. The mother was the good self and the daughter became similar to the good mother. As therapy proceeded, good and bad were integrated so that good and bad feelings were projected into the mother, and good object relations were integrated into her ego.

Sue's throwing about of the animals, people, and furniture showed her state of disintegration. As she worked through the fantasy of sadism and retaliation and experienced her sadness at possibly harming her mother, she could introject good objects and feel like a more complete person.

When projective identification was excessive, not only did she need to control the mother, but she had little energy left to generate speech to anyone else, particularly in situations such as classrooms, which make such demands on children.

She was incapable of taking back her projections and viewed the classroom as a dangerous place. She feared that if she spoke, her speech would be aggressive and that the teacher-mother, who could not or would not be controlled, would retaliate. Sue believed that the other children in the class would attack her if she was aggressive to their teacher-mother. Her response to this anxiety was to be silent in class and in school.

As treatment proceeded Sue began to make things as an act of reparation. This ensured in fantasy that her mother would not attack her in turn. She felt she repaired the mother by giving her the genitals of her brothers (the plasticene penises she created for the family that were later dumped into the toilet) and by the drawings and cut-out collages she made, and so she was able to lessen her control over her mother and her fears of retaliation. As the good mother was placed with the father and then with the daughter, Sue felt more whole and less frightened of people and her responses to them. Her fantasies became less sadistic and more reparative and nurturing, as seen in her drawings, which became less destructive and filled with "hearts."

CONCLUSION

Sometimes we hear that elective mutism as a symptom suddenly vanishes. In the few cases of this sort that I followed up, I have found that the child developed other problems. In two cases (aged 6 and 7) the mutism became reading difficulties (described as of psychological origin by a school psychologist); in two other cases, the children, aged 6, developed many somatic complaints (of a nonorganic origin) after they started to talk; in another case, a 10-year-old boy became very depressed and withdrawn, failing all his schoolwork after he started to talk outside of the home.

Elective mutism appears to be a distortion, at a point of crisis, of a basic process of psychic development. Each case will reveal its own special pattern of interconnection that links the child's experience of self, family, and outside world. Given a basic understanding of the source of the symptoms, we must respect these particularities and sensitively adjust our therapeutic approach, if we are to help such children.

REFERENCES

Anthony, E. J. (1977). Nonverbal and verbal systems of communication. *Psychoanalytic Study of the Child* 32:307–325. New Haven, CT: Yale University Press.

Blotcky, M. J., and Looney, J. G. (1980). A psychotherapeutic approach to silent children. *American Journal of Psychotherapy* 24(4):487–495.

Bradley, S., and Sloman, L. (1975). Elective mutism in immigrant families. *Journal of the American Academy of Child Psychiatry* 7:510–514.

Crema, J. E., and Kerr, J. M. (1978). Elective mutism: a child care case study. *Child Care Quarterly* 7(3):215–226.

Crisp, P. (1986). Projective identification: an attempt at clarification. *Journal of the Melanie Klein Society* 4(1):47–76.

Hesselman, S. (1983). Elective mutism in children 1877–1981. *Acta Paedopsychiatrica* 49:297–310.

Kaplan, S. L., and Escoll, P. (1973). Treatment of two silent adolescent girls. *Journal of the American Academy of Child Psychiatry* 12:59–72.

Meyers, S. V. (1984). Elective mutism in children: a family systems approach. *American Journal of Family Therapy* 12(4):39–45.

PART IV

PSYCHOPHARMACOLOGIC APPROACHES

10

ELECTIVE MUTISM AS A VARIANT OF SOCIAL PHOBIA

Bruce Black and Thomas W. Uhde

ELECTIVE MUTISM IS a psychiatric disorder of childhood characterized by persistent refusal to talk in one or more major social situations (including school) despite the ability to speak and comprehend spoken language. Children manifesting the disorder characteristically refuse to talk in school and to strangers. Although symptoms may be apparent from the preschool years, the disorder generally does not come to clinical attention until the child starts school. Transient manifestations of mutism after starting school are not uncommon. However, persistent forms of the disorder are rare (Brown and Lloyd 1975).

The term *elektiver Mutismus bei Kindern* was first used in the clinical literature in 1934 (Tramer 1934), although the symptom had been described and discussed many times as far back as the late nineteenth century (Hesselman 1983). Tramer's concept of the syndrome was of nonpsychotic children who spoke only to a small group of intimate acquaintances. From the earliest descriptions, shyness, timidity, and social withdrawal have been almost universally mentioned as characteristics of children with elective mutism.

Social phobia is an anxiety disorder characterized by a persistent fear of one or more social situations in which the person exposed to possible scrutiny by others fears that he or she may do something or act in a way that will be humiliating or embarrassing. Fear and avoidance of speaking in public or to strangers are among the most common symptoms reported by social phobics (Uhde et al. 1991). The disorder characteristically has its onset in childhood ("as far back as I can remember").

This chapter describes the case of a young girl with elective mutism associated with social anxiety who responded to treatment with fluoxetine, a medication shown to be effective in the treatment of social phobia (Black et al. 1992).

CASE PRESENTATION

Rebecca was a 12-year-old white girl who had never spoken a word in school. Before age 8, she had never spoken to anyone outside her immediate family. During the last several years, she had been able to speak freely to two close friends who did not attend her school but never spoke to children from her school, even when she encountered them away from school. She had a number of friends from school with whom she frequently spent time, including visiting one another's homes and going to shopping malls together. However, she had never spoken to these friends in person, although she did speak to them on the telephone. Her speech and language were entirely normal when she did speak.

Rebecca had told her mother that she was reluctant to talk because her voice sounded funny and she did not want others to hear it. She had always been very anxious and reticent to interact with nonfamily members and avoided all social interactions, including parties, using public bathrooms, and any interaction with strangers. When out with her mother in stores or other public settings, she insisted that her mother speak in a whisper for fear that she would draw attention to them if she spoke in a normal voice. She would play with her parents and siblings in their secluded backyard but never in their front yard where passersby might observe her. When her brother's playmates came to visit the home, she would retreat to her room for 24 to 36 hours at a time, refusing to come out even after the playmates had left. She had been fearful of eating in public and manifested symptoms of separation anxiety up to age 5 years. There was no history of school refusal.

Although she had never given an oral presentation or even responded verbally to questions in school, she had performed well academically. Standard achievement test scores were in the superior range, intelligence in the bright-normal range, and she consistently had high grades. Her teacher and school principal expressed a great deal of concern regarding her refusal to speak and increasing social avoidance but denied any other behavioral or emotional difficulties. In fact, her teacher described Rebecca as "an extremely well-adjusted student who does excellent work. Her only problem appears to be that she won't talk." Total score on the Connors' Teacher Questionnaire was zero (Connors 1985b). She was generally accepted by her classmates, to the extent that they would speak for her and explain to substitute teachers or other unfamiliar adults that she didn't talk. However, she had few friends, a very restricted scope of social activities, and was increasingly being ridiculed and teased by peers.

When brought for evaluation, Rebecca would not speak to or have any eye contact with the examiner. She willingly completed several symptom self-rating scales and on these scales acknowledged some mild-moderate social anxiety. However, many of her responses were internally inconsistent, contradicted her parents' reports, and did not appear to be valid. She insisted to her parents that there was not a problem, that she could speak if she wanted to but just didn't feel like it. The patient's mother was interviewed using the Anxiety Disorders Interview Schedule for children, Parent version (Silverman and Nelles 1988). She denied any specific signs or symptoms of mood disorders, appetite or sleep disturbance, simple phobias (except mild needle phobia), or obsessive-compulsive disorder. The Connors' Parent Symptom Questionnaire (Connors 1985a) showed an elevated score on the anxiety subscale. At the time of evaluation, Rebecca was one year postmenarche. Family psychiatric history was remarkable for mild public speaking anxiety in the father and a maternal history of childhood shyness.

Rebecca had been treated with outpatient psychotherapy for a year at age 5 to 6 years without benefit. At age 11, a school psychologist attempted a program of behavioral therapy, also without benefit.

A single-blind medication trial (with Rebecca and her parents blind) was recommended and accepted by the parents. No individual or family psychotherapy was provided. Although she initially refused to take medication, she later volunteered to her parents that she was willing to take medication if it was hidden in food and that she preferred to do this rather than not take medication. Thus, her mother did administer medication to her by mixing it into her food or drink. Rebecca was aware of this but pretended not to be. Prospective symptom severity and symptom change rating scales were completed by the parents on a weekly basis. Rebecca was treated with placebo for three weeks with no response, then with desipramine starting at 25 mg daily, increased over three weeks to 200 mg and continued for ten weeks. Because of the logistical difficulties of hiding the medication in her food, the dosage varied considerably from day to day within a range of 0 to 200 mg daily. Treatment was also complicated by her refusal to have an electrocardiogram or to have vital signs monitored in the clinic. Home vital sign monitoring was attempted, but results were unreliable. Her parents reported slight improvements in mood, minimally increased social interactions with peers, and decreased self-consciousness in public. She was able to speak with store clerks, which she had been unwilling to do previously, but continued to refuse to speak at school and with peers and to avoid social events such as parties.

Because of the minimal therapeutic change, the day-to-day variations in her dose, and the difficulty in maintaining appropriate medical monitoring, desipramine was tapered and discontinued at the beginning of the summer school vacation. She did not receive medication for one month and did not experience any changes in symptoms. She began receiving fluoxetine (parents were no longer blind) at 20 mg every other day for seven days, then 20 mg daily. She returned to school in the fall four weeks after she began receiving fluoxetine, and spoke freely with adults and peers. She gave oral reports in class without any apparent distress, volunteered oral responses to questions, and conversed freely with classmates in and out of the classroom. She attended school parties and dances without difficulty. After seven months, all of these gains were maintained, and her social communication and social interactions seemed to be entirely normal. However, she continued to refuse to speak with or establish any eye contact with her treating physician and in discussions with her parents continued to maintain that she had never had a problem with talking and had no need of medication. She did occasionally remark positively on the changes she had manifested but insisted medication had not played any role. She continued to refuse to agree to take medication or to acknowledge that she was knowingly taking it but very intentionally cooperated in drinking all her daily orange juice containing the "hidden" medication.

DISCUSSION

The commonly recommended forms of treatment for elective mutism have been individual psychodynamic psychotherapy, family therapy, and behavior therapy (Kratochwill 1981, Labbe and Williamson 1984, Laybourne 1989). Only one other case of pharmacologic treatment of elective mutism has been reported. In that case, a 7-year-old girl with a two-year history of elective mutism was successfully treated with phenelzine (Golwyn and Weinstock 1990). The girl had been shy and reportedly "froze with anxiety" when asked to speak to the psychiatrist. Family history was remarkable for panic disorder and alcoholism.

In the first English language description of elective mutism, Salfield and colleagues (1950) stated, "Elective mutism can be understood as a fixation at an early infantile level, on which an apprehended danger situation is met by a refusal to speak." Indeed, reluctance or refusal to speak is a frequently observed symptom of anxiety or apprehension of danger. It is a common manifestation of stranger anxiety in normal toddlers and preschool children. Remaining quiet and withdrawing are commonly observed signs of apprehension of danger in many animal species and have been observed as manifestations of anxiety like behaviors in a number of animal models of anxiety (Klein et al. 1987, Suomi 1986). Even normal, non–anxiety-disordered adults or children may remain quiet in frightening situations, particularly new social situations.

Similarly, since the earliest clinical descriptions of the syndrome, anxiety in the form of shyness, timidity, and social withdrawal has been universally mentioned as characteristic of the great majority of children with elective mutism (Brown and Lloyd 1975, Kolvin and Fundudis 1981, Pustrom and Speers 1964). Furthermore, a history of extreme shyness, timidity, overt social phobia or a history of childhood elective mutism is often reported in parents of elective mute children (Brown and Lloyd 1975, Pustrom and Speers 1964, Reed 1963, Salfield et al. 1950).

DSM-III-R (American Psychiatric Association, 1987) lists shyness, social isolation and withdrawal, clinging, compulsive traits, and school refusal as associated features of elective mutism, but anxiety disorder is not mentioned in the discussion of differential diagnosis. DSM-III-R states that in cases of elective mutism the refusal to talk is not a symptom of social phobia, but this is not a formal exclusion criteria for the diagnosis.

Elective mutism most often becomes manifest on starting school or preschool (Lesser-Katz 1986). In the only controlled, population-based study of elective mute children, Brown and Lloyd (1975) surveyed all 4½- to 5½-year-old children starting school in an English school district. Forty-two of 6,072 children (6.9 per 1,000) were not speaking in school after eight weeks. However, by twenty-four weeks, this number was down to fifteen, by thirty-two weeks to five, and by sixty-four weeks to one. Thus, transient elective mutism may be much more common than persistent mutism. They compared the forty-two children not speaking eight weeks after starting school with forty-two age- and sex-matched controls from the same population. Cases and controls were compared on a variety of developmental, demographic, family, and behavioral characteristics by means of school and home questionnaires completed between twenty-eight and thirty-two weeks after starting school (when most of the children were no longer mute). Cases were significantly more likely than controls to have one or both shy parents (51 percent versus 7 percent), to come from families who rarely went out together (37 percent versus 2 percent), and to have a sibling who had been mute (32 percent versus 15 percent). They were significantly more likely to stop an activity when the teacher approached (64 percent versus 0 percent), to avoid playing with other children (33 percent versus 2 percent), and were less likely to draw (26 percent versus 0 percent), go to the toilet (11 percent versus 0 percent), or approach the teacher's table (45 percent versus 2 percent).

All case series of elective mutism published in English (with more than ten subjects and with the gender of the subjects reported) were reviewed with regard to the gender distribution of the subjects. Of these cases, 143 were female and 75 were male, yielding a female:male sex ratio of 1.9:1 (Hayden 1980, Kolvin and Fundudis 1981, Parker et al. 1960, Wergeland 1979, Wilkins 1985, Wright 1968). Very few data are available regarding the sex ratio of anxiety disorders in children. However, one case series of children with avoidant disorder of childhood, which is the childhood analogue of social phobia, reported that sixteen of twenty-two cases seen were girls (F:M = 2.6:1) (Klein and Last 1989). Beidel (1991) reported a nonreferred cohort of eighteen children with social phobia, with a F:M ratio of 1.6:1. In contrast, among clinical samples of children with retarded speech development, the F:M ratio is generally in the range of 1:2-3 (Kolvin and Fundudis 1981).

If mutism is a common manifestation of anxiety, particularly social anxiety, and social anxiety is a universal characteristic of children with elective mutism, then is elective mutism simply a symptom of or variation of social phobia? The child presented here met the *DSM-III-R* diagnostic criteria for social phobia, and it seems more reasonable to regard her mutism as a manifestation of her social phobia rather than as a separate diagnosis. Many other cases of elective mutism in the clinical literature have been described with enough detail to say they appear to meet diagnostic criteria for social phobia.

It has been argued elsewhere that separation anxiety, when it occurs in children who have manifested a prepubertal onset of panic disorder, is more reasonably regarded as a developmental variant of agoraphobia, that is, as a constellation of symptoms (e.g., fear of not being able to contact a parent in the event of a panic attack) one might expect to see in an agoraphobic child, rather than as a separate diagnosis of separation anxiety disorder (Abelson and Alessi 1992, Black et al. 1990). Similarly, the syndrome of elective mutism as it is commonly described, that is, mutism when confronted by strangers or crowds (e.g., in school), may be no more than a developmental variant of social phobia, that is, a symptom one might expect to see in a social phobic school-age child.

Adult social phobics commonly avoid speaking in public or in new social situations. As they become more accustomed to a social situation, they are more likely to talk. Likewise, most children with elective mutism seem to be able to talk after they have had some time to become familiar with their teacher and classmates. Thus, elective mutism appears to be a symptom of social phobia in both children and adults. For developmental reasons it may be more common in social phobic children, although in social phobic adults it is less severe and more transient, and it is not likely to be labeled as elective mutism. Adults are more able to control their environments and to avoid situations where they are likely to be called on to speak. Again, this is analogous to the situation with panic disorder and separation anxiety disorder. The constellation of symptoms described as separation anxiety disorder also may be seen in persons with adult-onset panic disorder (but is generally less a focus of concern and treatment) and is generally not labeled as separation anxiety disorder.

A family history of shyness or other symptoms of social phobia were also present in our case and in many cases presented in the literature. Social phobia has been shown to have an increased prevalence in families of social phobia probands (Fyer et al. 1991). The familial overlap of elective mutism and social phobia would lend support to the construct validity of subsuming the syndrome of elective mutism within the diagnostic category of social phobia. Similarly, beneficial responses to phenelzine and fluoxetine, both of which have been shown to be effective in the treatment of social phobia, would also be supportive (Black et al. 1992, Liebowitz et al. 1988).

One additional clinical feature seen in this and other cases of elective mutism merits discussion. In the clinical literature, elective mute children are commonly described as stubborn, obstinate, and passive-aggressive, and these descriptors could apply to the child reported here. Rebecca's absolute refusal to ever acknowledge that her mutism was a problem, her extraordinary ambivalence about taking medication, and her continued refusal to speak to or have eye contact with her physician long after she was speaking comfortably elsewhere were all striking. Interestingly, other cases have been reported where symptoms resolve outside the treating clinician's office but the child continues to refuse to speak to the clinician (Elson et al. 1965, Mora et al. 1962, Pustrom and Speers 1964). Why do most elective mute children start speaking in school after a brief period (days to months) of adjustment, although others continue to refuse to speak even after many years? Personality features such as those described above play a role in the development or maintenance of elective mutism in children with social phobia, but this is no more than speculation at this time.

Other authors have also raised questions about the diagnostic classification of elective mutism (Kratochwill 1981, Wilkins 1985). Specifically, many authors have commented on the profound shyness noted in most patients with elective mutism and have argued that this supports its classification as a neurotic or emotional disorder. Wilkins retrospectively compared twenty-four elective mute children with twenty-four matched children diagnosed as suffering from emotional disorders and found few significant differences between the two groups. Likewise, others have suggested that elective mutism may be related to social phobia (Golwyn and Weinstock 1990) or to stranger anxiety (Lesser-Katz 1986). ICD-9-CM (*International Classification of Diseases*, 9th Revision, Clinical Modification) includes elective mutism (313.23) as a subcategory of sensitivity, shyness, and social withdrawal disorder.

There have been no controlled treatment studies of elective mutism. Many cases seem to resolve or to show improvement over time, although others seem to endure and to be resistant to multiple treatment interventions. It is not clear whether treatment has any effect on outcome. One small study compared long-term outcome in six treated children and five untreated children and concluded that the untreated children actually fared better than did the treated children (Wergeland 1979). This is only the second reported case of pharmacologic treatment. In both cases, the symptoms were long standing and had shown no response to nonpharmacologic treatments. Dramatic improvements were associated with phamacologic treatment. Furthermore, in the case presented here there had been no response to placebo treatment and minimal response to treatment with desipramine.

CONCLUSIONS

A case of elective mutism associated with social phobia in a 12-year-old girl, responsive to treatment with fluoxetine, has been presented. It has been argued that elective mutism may be a manifestation of social phobia rather than a separate diagnostic entity.

The best nosological classification for the syndrome of elective mutism cannot be reliably decided on the basis of currently available evidence. However, it frequently may be a manifestation of social phobia. Appropriate diagnosis when this is the case may facilitate more effective treatment. Further clinical and population-based surveys of children refusing to speak in school, using standardized diagnostic interviews, follow-up studies, family studies, neurobiological assessments, and assessment of response to different treatment modalities may provide more useful information to ascertain the relationship of this syndrome to social phobia and to other diagnostic categories.

Although the efficacy of phamacologic treatment for elective mutism has not been established, a trial of fluoxetine or phenelzine should be considered in cases where the symptoms are long standing, causing significant impairment, and where other forms of treatment have not been successful.

REFERENCES

Abelson, J. L., and Alessi, N. E. (1992). Discussion of child panic revisited. *Journal of the American Academy of Child and Adolescent Psychiatry* 31:114–116.

American Psychiatric Association. (1987). *Diagnostic and Statistical Manual of Mental Disorders, Third Edition, Revised (DSM-III-R)*. Washington, DC: American Psychiatric Association.

Beidel, D. C. (1991). Social phobia and overanxious disorder in school-age children. *Journal of the American Academy of Child and Adolescent Psychiatry* 30(4):545–552.

Black, B., Robbins, D. R., and Uhde, T. W. (1990). Does panic disorder exist in childhood? *Journal of the American Academy of Child and Adolescent Psychiatry* 29:834–835.

Black, B., Uhde, T. W., and Tancer, M. E. (1992). Fluoxetine for treatment of social phobia. *Journal of Clinical Psychopharmacology* 12:293–295.

Brown, J. B., and Lloyd, H. (1975). A controlled study of children not speaking at school. *Journal of the Association of Workers for the Maladjusted Child* 3:49–63.

Connors, C. K. (1985a). Parent symptom questionnaire. *Psychopharmacological Bulletin* 21:816–822.

———— (1985b). Teacher questionnaire. *Psychopharmacological Bulletin* 21:823–827.

Elson, A., Pearson, C., Jones, C. D., and Schumacher, E. (1965). Follow-up study of childhood elective mutism. *Archives of General Psychiatry* 13:182–187.

Fyer, A. J., Mannuzza, S., Chapman, T., et al. (1991). *A family study of social phobia and panic disorder*. Paper presented at the annual meeting of the American Psychiatric Association. New Orleans, LA, May.

Golwyn, D. H., and Weinstock, R. C. (1990). Phenelzine treatment of elective mutism. *Journal of Clinical Psychiatry* 51:384–385.

Hayden, T. L. (1980). Classification of elective mutism. *Journal of the American Academy Child Psychiatry* 19:118–133.

Hesselman, S. (1983). Elective mutism in children 1877–1981. *Acta Paedopsychiatrica* 49:297–310.

Klein, E., Marangos, P. J., Montgomery, P., et al. (1987). Adenosine receptor alterations in nervous pointer dogs: a preliminary report. *Clinical Neuropharmacology* 10:462–469.

Klein, R. G., and Last, C. G. (1989). *Anxiety Disorders in Children*. Newbury Park, CA: Sage.

Kolvin, I., and Fundudis, T. (1981). Elective mute children: psychological development and background factors. *Journal of Child Psychology and Psychiatry* 22:219–232.

Kratochwill, T. R. (1981). *Selective Mutism: Implications for Research and Treatment*. Hillsdale, NJ: Erlbaum.

Labbe, E. E., and Williamson, D. A. (1984). Behavioral treatment of elective mutism. *Clinical Psychology Review* 4:273–292.

Laybourne, P. C. (1989). Treatment of elective mutism. In *American Psychiatric Association: Treatments of Psychiatric Disorders: A Task Force Report of the American Psychiatric Association*, vol. 1, pp. 762–771. Washington, DC: American Psychiatric Association.

Lesser-Katz, M. (1986). Stranger reaction and elective mutism in young children. *American Journal of Orthopsychiatry* 56:458–469.

Liebowitz, M. R., Gorman, J. M., Fyer, A. J., et al. (1988). Pharmacotherapy of social phobia: an interim report of a placebo-controlled comparison of phenelzine and atenolol. *Journal of Clinical Psychiatry* 49:252–257.

Mora, G., DeVault, S., and Schopler, E. (1962). Dynamics and psychotherapy of identical twins with elective mutism. *Journal of Child Psychology and Psychiatry* 7:41–52.

Parker, E. B., Olsen, T. F., and Throckmorton, M. C. (1960). Social casework with elementary school children who do not talk in school. *Social Work* 5:64–70.

Pustrom, E., and Speers, R. W. (1964). Elective mutism in children. *Journal of the American Academy of Child Psychiatry* 3:287–297.

Reed, G. F. (1963). Elective mutism in children: a reappraisal. *Journal of Child Psychology and Psychiatry* 4:99–107.

Salfield, D. J., Lond, B. S., and Dusseldorn, M. D. (1950). Observations on elective mutism in children. *Journal of Mental Science* 96:1024–1032.

Silverman, W. K., and Nelles, W. B. (1988). The anxiety disorders interview schedule for children. *Journal of the American Academy of Child and Adolescent Psychiatry* 27:772–778.

Suomi, S. J. (1986). Anxiety-like disorders in young nonhuman primates. In *Anxiety Disorders of Childhood*, ed. R. Gittelman, pp. 1–23. New York: Guilford.

Tramer, M. (1934). Elektiver Mutismus bei Kindern. *Zeitschrift fur Kinderpsveiniaz* 1:30–35.

Uhde, T. W., Tancer, M. E., Black, B., and Brown, T. M. (1991). Phenomenology and neurobiology of social phobia: comparison with panic disorder. *Journal of Clinical Psychiatry* 52:31–40.

Wergeland, H. (1979). Elective mutism. *Acta Psychiatrica Scandinavica* 59:216–226.

Wilkins, R. (1985). A comparison of elective mutism and emotional disorders in children. *Behavioral Journal of Psychiatry* 146:198–203.

Wright. H. L. (1968). A clinical study of children who refuse to talk in school. *Journal of the American Academy of Child Psychiatry* 7:603–617.

11

PHENELZINE TREATMENT OF ELECTIVE MUTISM: A CASE REPORT

*Daniel H. Golwyn and
Ronda C. Weinstock*

ELECTIVE MUTISM AS defined by *DSM-III-R* is a disorder of childhood characterized by a persistent refusal to talk in one or more major social situations, including school, despite the ability to comprehend spoken language and to speak. It is a rare, often disabling condition with no known cause or cure. The *DSM-III-R* states that the mutism is not a symptom of social phobia, but excessive shyness is an associated feature of mutism. Most authors comment on the anxiety and profound shyness of the majority of children diagnosed as electively mute (Lesser-Katz 1986, Wilkins 1985), but the relationship of elective mutism to the anxiety disorders and social phobia has been neglected in the literature.

The treatment described by most researchers has been some form of behavior therapy, individual therapy, or family therapy. There is no treatment of choice, and one study on long-term follow-up found that the untreated patients were better adjusted than those who received treatment (Wergeland 1979). Most authors do, however, agree on the importance of early intervention (Lesser-Katz

1986, Wergeland 1979). On the basis of the reported success of monoamine oxidase inhibitors in the treatment of social phobia in adults (Liebowitz et al. 1988), the reports that these drugs are well tolerated in children (Kelly et al. 1970, Zametkin et al. 1985), our own unpublished observations that patients taking phenelzine become garrulous, and the expectation that phenelzine's dopaminergic effect might promote social engagement (Liebowitz et al. 1987), we administered phenelzine to a child who fulfilled *DSM-III-R* criteria for elective mutism and had associated shyness.

CASE REPORT

CASE 1

Mary, a 7-year-old white girl, had a two-year history of mutism outside her family. She spoke to her parents and sister without articulatory difficulties at home but was mute at school and with outsiders. Four months of behavioral psychotherapy and one month of treatment with the dopaminergic agent amantadine (200 mg/day) had failed. Past medical history was noncontributory. Mary had no developmental delays, childhood phobias, or conduct disorders. She had always been shy, but she did not avoid school or social functions. She had a playmate but did not converse with her. Her mother had abused alcohol and her father had had panic disorder that responded to phenelzine.

Mary presented as a bright, anxious, cooperative, petite (weight = 22 kg [49 lb], height = 123 cm [4 ft 1 in]) child who separated easily from her parents in the waiting room. When asked to speak, she froze with anxiety and remained mute. Her IQ was above average on the Wechsler Intelligence Scale for Children–Revised. Results of a CBC, blood chemistries, and thyroid studies were normal.

After instructing the parents about diet and medication warnings, treatment with phenelzine 7.5 mg t.i.d. (one-half of a 15-mg tablet t.i.d.) was started (total daily dose of 22.5 mg or 1 mg/kg). The dose was gradually increased to a maximum of 60 mg/day at 15 weeks. At six weeks, while receiving 37.5 mg/day, Mary began to talk more freely to her parents outside the home. Her appetite increased and mild constipation resulting from treatment was controlled with psyllium hydrophilic mucilloid. At 12 weeks, at a dose of 52.5 mg/day, she began conversing at day-care. At 16 weeks, when school reopened, Mary spoke freely to teachers, children, and both authors. Although her blood pressure decreased after exercise, Mary was never symptomatic of postural hypotension or oversedation. At 18 weeks, her weight was 30 kg (67 lb) and her height was 126 cm (4 ft 2 in). Results of subsequent laboratory tests were normal. The phenelzine dose was tapered and withdrawn by week 24. Five months later the mutism still had not recurred and Mary never explained her silence.

DISCUSSION

We believe our patient's response to phenelzine is the first reported case of a successful pharmacologic treatment of elective mutism. Her response to a pharmacologic treatment for social phobia, her family history of panic disorder, and the shyness and anxiety reported in the elective mutism literature raise nosologic questions about elective mutism and its relationship to social phobia and the anxiety disorders.

Questions may arise regarding the best diagnostic label for our patient. However, before treatment she was mute, an object of ridicule, unable to take oral examinations, and being considered for placement in an emotionally handicapped class. Whatever we label her condition, she spoke after treatment with phenelzine. Our approach follows the suggestion of van Praag and colleagues (1987) to focus on a functional approach to psychopathologic behaviors rather than on conventional diagnosis. Patients who are labeled as shy, anxious, depressed, avoidant, socially phobic, or electively mute may all be overly reticent. Regardless of nosologic ambiguities, treating this particular psychopathologic behavior with phenelzine might prove fruitful. In these conditions, phenelzine may induce increased speech

as well as decrease social anxiety. We can speculate that dopaminergic systems may regulate talkativeness as well as movement and activity in such diverse conditions as akinetic mutism, Parkinson's
disease, cocainism, bipolar disorder, schizophrenia, social phobia, and
elective mutism.

Drug names: amantadine (Symmetrel), phenelzine (Nardil).

REFERENCES

Kelly, D., Guirguis, W., Frommer, E., et al. (1970). Treatment of
    phobic states with antidepressants: a retrospective study of 246
    patients. *British Journal of Psychiatry* 116:387–398.
Lesser-Katz, M. (1986). Stranger reaction and elective mutism in
    young children. *American Journal of Orthopsychiatry* 56:458–469.
Liebowitz, M. R., Campeas, R., and Hollander, E. (1987). MAOIs:
    impact on social behavior (letter). *Psychiatry Research* 22:89–90.
Liebowitz, M. R., Gorman, J. M., Fyer, A. J., et al. (1988).
    Pharmacotherapy of social phobia: an interim report of a pla-
    cebo-controlled comparison of phenelzine and atenolol. *Journal
    of Clinical Psychiatry* 49:252–257.
van Praag, H. M., Kahn, P. S., Asnis, G. M., et al. (1987).
    Denosologization of biological psychiatry or the specificity of
    5-HT disturbances in psychiatric disorders. *Journal of Affective
    Disorders* 13:1–8.
Wergeland, H. (1979). Elective mutism. *Acta Psychiatrica Scandinavica*
    59:218–228.
Wilkins, R. (1985). A comparison of elective mutism and emotional
    disorders in children. *British Journal of Psychiatry* 146:198–203.
Zametkin, A., Rapoport, J. L., Murphy, D. L., et al. (1985). Treat-
    ment of hyperactive children with monoamine oxidase inhibi-
    tors, I: clinical efficacy. *Archives of General Psychiatry* 42:962–
    966.

PART V

GROUP AND FAMILY THERAPY

12

ELECTIVE MUTISM
IN CHILDREN:
A FAMILY SYSTEMS APPROACH

Susan V. Meyers

Silence is one great art of conversation.

Hazlitt (1837)

SILENT BEHAVIOR AND its syntax have remained somewhat of a mystery to psychotherapists as well as a source of discomfort and frustration. One type of silent behavior that psychotherapists may encounter is *elective mutism*, a term used to describe the rare behavior of children who possess the ability to talk but choose to remain silent.

The definition and terminology used to describe such individuals have been expanded as knowledge and studies of these children grow. Reporting of electively mute behavior dates back to 1877, when Kussmaul used the term *aphasia voluntaria*, or "voluntary mutism," to refer to mentally sound persons who force themselves into mutism for reasons they refuse to disclose. Tramer (1934) was the first to describe this condition under the term *elective mutism*, referring to children whose muteness was usually selective—most often the child spoke normally to the immediate family within the confines of his or her home, but was nonverbal with peers and teachers in school or in the world generally. Salfield and colleagues (1950) observed some commonalities in elective mutism: (1) its onset occurs between 3 and 5 years of age, (2) there is usually no mental defect, (3) there is often a familial factor, (4) it is resistant to treatment, (5) there are possible somatic psychological or compound traumas. Elson and colleagues (1965) add another dimension to the temporal origin of the symptom. Elective mutism is first manifested when the child separates from the family to attend school. School refusal or mild school phobia may occur. There is agreement in the field that the term *elective mutism* excludes all other forms of mutism, including mental retardation, schizophrenia, hysterical aphonia, aphasia, and hearing loss as provocative of silence.

PREVALENCE OF ELECTIVE MUTISM

Elective mutism in children is a relatively rare symptom, and as a result, little attention has been devoted to exploring its incidence. Bradley and Sloman (1975) have obtained statistical validation for their clinical impressions that there is an increased occurrence of electively mute behavior in children from immigrant families. The authors used a school survey and questionnaires to study children in Toronto, Canada, who ranged in grade from kindergarten through grade eight. In the total sample of 6,865 children, twenty-six exhibited electively mute behavior, twenty-three of whom were from immigrant families, and three of whom were from English-speaking families. (This difference is significant at .001.) Twenty of the mute children were in the kindergarten population. Bradley and Sloman concluded that elective mutism is definitely more likely to develop in children from immigrant families.

TYPES OF ELECTIVE MUTISM

Hayden (1980) classified sixty-eight elective mutes into four basic types: (1) symbiotic mutism, (2) speech phobic mutism, (3) reactive mutism, (4) passive-aggressive mutism. Symbiotic mutism, the most common type, showed a strong symbiotic relationship with a caregiver, usually (84 percent) the mother. In spite of a clinging, shy exterior, the child was manipulative and negativistic toward controlling situations and adults. Speech phobic mutism, the least common type was characterized by a fear of hearing one's own voice. Hayden postulated that family secrets might be revealed and that the child would feel unable to control his or her speech about such matters. Reactive mutes were typed by the fact that a single or series of traumatic events precipitated their silence. Examples included children who had been raped, or had experienced a death in the family, or had suffered mouth or throat injuries. In passive-aggressive mutism, silence was seen as a weapon, expressing hostility by a defiant refusal to speak. The dynamics of this behavior revealed the child as a family scapegoat. Such children were described as strong-willed and their mutism seen as a choice of something the child could manage and use to manipulate the less controllable world. Commonalities to all groups included physical tensions, rigidity, fearfulness, phobias, flattened affect, and considerable pathology in the family.

Hayden's classifications and her descriptions have provided a useful structure that has led to a better understanding of elective mutes and can assist in determining a suitable treatment plan. Bearing in mind Hayden's framework, the therapist needs to be cognizant of possible overlap in the categories as well as the individual differences that every elective mute and his or her family present.

CHARACTERISTICS OF ELECTIVE MUTISM FAMILIES

A recent trend is to study the kinds of families that produce electively mute children. Progress is being made in identifying behavior patterns common in such families. It is hoped that an enumeration of the similar characteristics, assembled from the literature (1960–1983) and the author's clinical experience, offers a family profile that will foster an understanding of the family system and aid in the formulation of treatment plans. The primary characteristics and their descriptions are:

1. Symbiosis (Goll 1979, Hayden 1980, Mora et al. 1962, Pustrom and Speers 1964)
2. Suspiciousness of outside world (Goll 1979, Parker et al. 1960)
3. Fear of strangers (Goll 1979, Parker et al. 1960)
4. Language difficulties—often experienced in immigrant families (Bradley and Sloman 1975)
5. Marital disharmony (Goll 1979, Meijer 1979, Pustrom and Speers 1964)
6. Mutism modeling (Goll 1979)
7. Strong tensions in family (Elson et al. 1965, Hayden 1980)
8. Extreme shyness (Meijer 1979)

SYMBIOSIS

The elective mutist has an intense attachment to another family member, most often the mother. This close relationship reflects an interdependency between the parent and child. Both feel that they cannot survive without the other, and participate in a symbiotic process that prohibits and interferes with individual growth and development. The symbiotic relationship is often threatened when a child first separates from home, as when the child enters school for the first time. The elective mutist's silence may in part stem from a loyalty to the symbiotic partner and/or family, for example, "I will not reveal family secrets. I won't tell." Hayden (1980) believed that the symbiotic mutist was one of distinct type of elective mutism.

SUSPICIOUSNESS OF THE OUTSIDE WORLD

Elective mutes have been taught by their families that the outer world is an unsafe and dangerously forbidding place. The condition was found to be more prevalent in immigrant families (Bradley and Sloman 1975) where differences in customs, language, and financial status may result in a distrust of a diverse culture. Family members may feel alienated and isolated. Furthermore, elective mutist families highly value loyalty to their family system, which may interfere with acceptance of their outside environment as a trusted resource. This loyalty factor may or may not be related to cultural status.

FEAR OF STRANGERS

The elective mutist family considers people outside of the family system as a threat to their well-being. Parents and grandparents have often modeled silence as a reaction to strangers (Parker et al. 1960). The electively mute child is, in part, emulating the parental behavior that he or she observes, and also expressing loyalty to his or her family, for example, "It is not safe or loyal to speak in front of strangers outside the confines of the family."

LANGUAGE DIFFICULTIES

Elective mutism is definitely more likely to develop in children of immigrant families (Bradley and Sloman 1975). Such families often experience communication problems related to the hardship of learning a new language. Unfortunately, language gaps often represent a barrier to cultural adjustment.

MARITAL DISHARMONY

The parents of elective mutists often feel alienated from one another. Communication skills are usually poor, or if previously present, have later deteriorated. Meijer (1979) describes the mothers of elective mutists as resentful toward the fathers. The troubled marital relationship often triangulates a child to absorb the stress. Parent and child coalitions form and the elective mutist serves as a shuttlecock of marital dissatisfaction.

MUTIST MODELING

Silent behavior is often practiced by one or both parents as a way of coping with stress. The silence is sometimes used as a weapon in the marital relationship and serves as a way to avoid difficulties in the marriage. Furthermore, this silent behavior is often modeled, condoned, and reinforced in such family systems. The child learns a silent way of relating and/or retreating.

STRONG TENSIONS IN THE FAMILY

Marital dissatisfaction, lack of communication in the family system, culturally related assimilation problems, and overall denial of the existence of problems represent overwhelming internal stress in elective mutist families.

EXTREME SHYNESS

Language difficulties, cultural gaps, and a family condoning of silent behavior add to the fears of mutist family members in making statements and verbal commitments or expressing their feelings.

SUMMARY

The above characteristics indicate the family's involvement in the complex symptomatology of the elective mute. Elective mutism has been shown to be based in parent mutist modeling, family cultural tradition, symbiotic attachment, separation anxiety, and poor marital adjustment. The family constitutes a tightly knit social system where significant emotional exchanges are self-contained and where there is a generalized fear of strangers and the outside world.

TREATMENT OF ELECTIVE MUTISM

While speech therapy (Adams and Glasner 1954) was given some attention as a treatment mode between 1940 and 1960, it has received little notice in recent literature. During the past 10 years, most of the major studies have utilized one or more of the following approaches: psychoanalytic (Ambrosino and Alessi 1979, Chethik 1973, Youngerman 1979), individual psychotherapy (Ruzicka and Sackin

1974, Wergeland 1979), and behavior modification (Kratochwill 1981, Nash et al. 1979, Richards and Hansen 1978, Sanok and Streifel 1979). Rosenberg and Lindblad (1978) utilized behavior modification techniques in a family context.

FAMILY SYSTEMS APPROACH

Since family systems theory in general represents relatively new thinking, it is understandable that its application to the rare condition of elective mutism would take time to be reported in journals. Therefore, there is a paucity of information on family therapy approaches to such a symptomatology.

Pustrom and Speers (1964) concluded, "The symptom of elective mutism is a compromise expression of family conflict" (p. 296). In a study of three electively mute children and their families, they found an intense mother–child dependency, marital discord, and conflicts relating to talking. Anxiety about verbalizing primarily involved fears of revealing "family secrets." Their therapeutic recommendations were family oriented, with particular attention paid to the marital relationship and the mother–child dependency needs. The electively mute child was seen as reacting to family disturbance and his or her therapy involved dealing with his aggressive impulses and the dependency on the mother. Pustrom and Speers recommended employing a family approach when confronted with an electively mute child.

Goll (1979) broadened the understanding of elective mutism by describing a similar role structure and subculture in such families. He presented ten case studies and found that each family consisted of individuals playing four roles:

1. Elective mutist (EM), the identified patient
2. Mutist model (MM), a family member imitated
3. Symbiotic partner (SP), a family member closely tied to and dependent on the identified patient
4. Ghetto leader (GH), a person or persons who distrust society and its official representatives

The EM child from such a ghetto family is confronted with a crisis situation when starting kindergarten. The child is among "foreigners" and must talk to strangers, which may mean being a traitor to the ghetto. One desirable treatment strategy would be for the therapist to break down the family's distrust of the outer milieu. This process was seen as extremely difficult because the therapist was viewed as representative of alien society. Goll (1979) stated that although many authors have tried forms of behavior modification with varying success, the prognosis for elective mutism seemed to depend on contact between home and therapist. Without parental support, the disturbed family patterns would persist and the mutism could recur or in some cases worsen into total mutism.

CASE REPORT

The application of a family systems theoretical framework to the treatment of elective mutism is illustrated by the case of the W Family, a Chinese-American family, and their 5-year-old daughter, Gloria. This case from the author's clinical practice is demonstrative of elective mutism as a family problem that expressed family conflict.

Understanding why Gloria elected to become mute facilitated and, in part, determined the course of therapy. Gloria's mother, Althea, was the mutist model from whom Gloria learned silence as a way of dealing with anxiety and of manipulating others' behaviors. Althea and Gloria were symbiotic partners who needed each other to survive. David, Gloria's 7-year-old brother, was the sibling partner (who represented male Chinese perfection) against whom she exhibited anger and hostility. Gloria's father, Len, was the "ghetto leader" to whom Goll refers, and through whom all communications in the family went.

The family was further characterized by extreme shyness, suspiciousness of the outside world, fear of strangers, language difficulties, marital disharmony, and strong tensions. Other symptomatology present in the W family were Gloria's gender confusion, separation anxiety, and acting out behavior at home; David's severe asthma; Althea's depression; and Len's debilitating headaches. Gloria was the family scapegoat and primary symptom bearer. The various roles described resulted in destructive patterns that prevented growth. The root of the electively mute behavior lay in dysfunctional family relationships.

Gloria and Althea's symbiotic relationship related, in part, to a hostile and disappointing relationship between Len and Althea. Working on and improving their marital relationship was a vital therapeutic strategy. This intervention dealt with symbiosis between parent and child indirectly and without being an immediate threat to their closeness. As marital satisfaction grew, symbiosis was no longer necessary to maintain equilibrium in the family. Althea's growing relationship with the therapist also reduced her need to maintain the mother–child dependency.

Work with the W family revealed that Gloria's silence represented, in part, intense loyalty to her traditional Chinese family. She was not going to reveal any family secrets in the perceived unfriendly environment of a diverse American society. Gloria's therapy included play therapy meetings at her home and at the therapist's office, as well as sessions with her along with other members of her family.

Including the family in therapy and dealing with their conflicts as well assured an overall improvement of family functioning because each member was aware of and involved in one another's changes. Growth in the W family individually, in the marital relationship, and the sibling subsystem served to maintain the homeostatic balance in the family system as a whole.

The result of therapy, including three follow-up visits over a span of four years, reveals Gloria electively verbal and identified with her feminine gender, Althea functioning as an independent woman with a voice in the family, Len without headaches, Althea and Len communicating and valuing their relationship, and David without asthmatic symptoms. The crucial element, as viewed by the author, in the successful outcome of the case of Gloria and her family was due to the utilization of family systems theory as a way of conceptualizing the problem and as a basis for forming a therapeutic relationship with all of the family members (Meyers 1982).

COMMENT

The salient findings resulting from a review of recent literature and the author's clinical experience are as follows:

1. Elective mutism is a relatively rare symptom. Its prevalence among elementary school children in Canada is approximately 1 in 264.
2. The kindergarten population comprises the highest percentage of elective mutes.
3. Elective mutism is more likely to occur in children from immigrant families.
4. Elective mutism excludes all other forms of mutism, such as mental retardation, schizophrenia, hysterical aphonia, aphasia, and hearing loss.
5. Four basic types of elective mutism are symbiotic mutism, speech phobic mutism, reactive mutism, and passive-aggressive mutism.
6. Characteristics of elective mutists' families include symbiosis, suspiciousness of the outside world, fear of strangers, marital disharmony, mutist modeling, strong tensions in the family, and extreme shyness.
7. The family dynamics integral in the symptomatology of elective mutism make it advisable to include the family when formulating a treatment plan.

In view of the above findings, it is recommended that the present concept of elective mutism be extended to include the family. The broader position might be stated as follows:

Elective mutism refers to a relatively rare behavior pattern in which children who possess age-appropriate speech choose to remain silent, speaking only to self-selected persons. The small circle of intimates to whom the elective mutist speaks is usually composed of family members, relatives, or close friends. This selective refusal to speak is independent of intellectual endowment and/or neurotic status. Elective mutism is a symptom of a family problem that expresses family conflict and is embedded in family dynamics.

This definition more completely and accurately describes the role of the silent but eloquent symptom. Another factor, the importance of which should not be underestimated when referring to the family in an expanded view of elective mutism, is that it would influence a therapist's thinking about the problem and in part determine his or her approach.

Since elective mutism is an uncommon symptom, most therapists encountering it for the first time will seek information to help decide the process by which therapy should proceed. In attempting to make this decision the therapist has several options from which to choose. One option would be to refer the case to a therapist who specializes in the family systems approach. Another would be to assume his or her particular child-oriented approach while recognizing the importance of family dynamics. A third might be to use a family therapist as a resource coordinator for the child's treatment and services. This family therapist would serve as an appropriate referral source, contact for the child's teacher, support for the parents, and family systems educator for the clinician working with the case. In addition to assuring work with the family, the resource coordinator would draw together the various disciplines, including speech therapist, behavior modification specialist, psychotherapist, and educator.

In conclusion, elective mutists and their families offer the family therapist an important new clinical population with which to work, and, furthermore, give the therapist the opportunity for a personally and professionally satisfying experience. This chapter introduced the clinician to the significance of the family dynamics present within the symptom of elective mutism.

Not able to speak, but unable to be silent.
Epicharmus, ca. 550 B.C.

ACKNOWLEDGMENT

The author acknowledges the assistance of Dr. Chris Hatcher of the Langley-Porter Institute, University of California, San Francisco.

REFERENCES

Adams, H., and Glasner, P. (1954). Emotional involvements in some forms of mutism. *Journal of Speech and Hearing Disorders* 19:59–69.

Ambrosino, S., and Alessi, M. (1979). Elective mutism: fixation and the double bind. *American Journal of Psychoanalysis* 39(3):251–256.

Bradley, S., and Sloman, L. (1975). Elective mutism in immigrant families. *Journal of American Academy of Child Psychiatry* 1:510–514.

Chethik, M. (1973). Amy: the intensive treatment of an elective mute. *Journal of the American Academy of Psychiatry* 1:482–498.

Elson, A., Pearson, C., Jones, C., and Schumacher, E. (1965). Follow-up study of childhood elective mutisim. *Archives of General Psychiatry* 13:192–197.

Epicharmus. (C. 500 B.C.). *Fragments.* Leben and Schriften des Koers Epicharmos. Nebts einer fragmentens ammlung, by August Otto Friedrich Lorenz. Berlin, 1864.

Goll, K. (1979). Role structure and subculture in families of elective mutists. *Family Process* 18(1):55–56.

Hayden, R. (1980). Classification of elective mutism. *Journal of the American Academy of Child Psychiatry* 19(7):621–630.

Hazlitt, W. (1837). *Characteristics: In the Manner of Rochefoucault's Maxims.* London: J. Templeman.

Kratochwill, T. (1981). *Selective Mutism: Implications for Research and Treatment.* Hillsdale, NJ: Erlbaum.

Kussmaul, A. (1877). In Von Misch, A. (1952). Elektiver mutisimus im kindersalter. *Zeitschrift Fuer Kinder Psychiatrie* A:49–87.

Meijer, A. (1979). Elective mutism in children. *Israel Annals of Psychiatry and Related Disciplines* 17(2):93–100.

Meyers, S. (1982). *Elective mutism in children: a family systems approach.* Doctoral Dissertation, California Graduate School of Marital and Family Therapy.

Mora, G., Devault, S., and Schopler, E. (1962). Dynamics and psychotherapy of identical twins with elective mutism. *Journal of Child Psychoanalysis and Psychiatry* 3:41–52.

Nash, R., Thorpe, H., Andrews, M., and Davis, K. (1979). A management program for elective mutism. *Psychology in the Schools* 16(2):246–253.

Parker, E., Olsen, T., and Throckmorton, M. (1960). Social casework with elementary school children who do not talk in school. *Social Work* 5:64–70.

Pustrom, E., and Speers, R. (1964). Elective mutism in children. *Journal of the American Academy of Child Psychiatry* 3:287–297.

Richards, S., and Hansen, M. (1978). A further demonstration of the efficacy of stimulus fading treatment of elective mutism. *Journal of Behavior Therapy and Experimental Psychiatry* 9:57–60.

Rosenberg J., and Lindblad, M. (1978). Behavior therapy in a family context: treating elective mutism. *Family Process* 17:77–82.

Ruzicka, B., and Sackin, H. (1974). Elective mutism: the impact of the patient's silent detachment upon the therapist. *Journal of the American Academy of Child Psychiatry* 13:551–561.

Salfield, D., Lond, B., and Dusseldorf, M. (1950). Observations on elective mutism in children. *Journal of Mental Sciences* 96:1024–1032.

Sanok, R., and Streifel, S. (1979). Elective mutism: generalization of verbal responding across people and settings. *Behavior Therapy* 10(3):357–371.

Tramer, M. (1934). Elektiver mutism bei kindern. *Zeitschrift Kinderpathisher* 1:30–35.

Wergeland, H. (1979). Elective mutism. *Acta Psychiatrica Scandinavica* 59:218–228.

Youngerman, J. (1979). The syntax of silence: electively mute therapy. *International Review of Psychoanalyis* 6(3):283–295.

13

GROUP TREATMENT FOR ELECTIVE MUTE CHILDREN

James A. Bozigar and
Ruth Aguilar Hansen

ELECTIVE MUTISM, A condition most frequently occurring in children, manifests the following diagnosed criteria: (1) refusal to talk in almost all social situations, including school; (2) ability to comprehend spoken language and to speak; and (3) absence of any organic mental or physical disorder that causes the problem (*DSM-III*; American Psychiatric Association 1980). Various theories have been proposed to explain the cause of elective mutism. Halpern and colleagues (1971) have done an extensive study and have recognized the following as being possible causes of the disorder: (1) low self-esteem and poor social skills; (2) trauma during critical developmental stages; (3) uncertain, insecure home life; (4) emotional disturbance that is not attributed to another mental disorder; and (5) neurotic behavior as a result of family dysfunction. In addition, elective mutism has also been associated with such difficulties as school phobia, disfluent speech, separation, anxiety, resistive behavior, compulsivity, and enuresis (Halpern et al. 1971).

Research indicates that a variety of treatment modalities—ranging from inpatient hospitalization with aversion therapy to outpatient individual psychotherapy—have been tried for curing elective mutism (Browne et al. 1963, Chapin and Corcoran 1947, Chethik 1973, Halpern et al. 1971, Mora et al. 1962, Morris 1953, Nolan and Pence 1970, Parker et al. 1960, Reid et al. 1967, Straughan et al. 1965, Weinberger et al. 1967). The authors did not find in the literature any mention of group treatment, which appears to be a unique approach to helping these children overcome their disorder.

This chapter outlines both broad and specific treatment issues concerning elective mute children. A group treatment modality is presented, and its successes, limitations, and failures are noted with recommendations for avoiding pitfalls in treatment. Issues of cooperation with schools, families, and community organizations are also addressed with respect to this debilitating mental health problem.

GROUP APPROACH

At La Frontera Community Mental Health Center in South Tucson, Arizona, group therapy was undertaken when four elective mute children were referred by their schools for treatment. Although group membership was small, it is the opinion of the authors that elective mute clients demand intensive and structured interaction. To accomplish this, two therapists are essential. The group at La Frontera was conducted by the authors, a male and a female therapist, a setup that structured the interaction and also helped the children expand their relationship with adults of both sexes. Coleadership allowed the therapists to assess the children's reaction to different adults and enabled them to evaluate the children's use of mutism in controlling their relationships with adults.

The group met for 60 minutes weekly, and additional individual sessions were held as necessary. As the children progressed, it was critical to increase the number of contacts, which took place at the schools and consisted of an intensive, week-long desensitization period.

The length of treatment varied with each child, from two months to one year. Many factors influenced the length of treatment, including the therapists' workload, the children's attendance, and most significantly, the schools' cooperation. This latter issue has a tremendous impact on length of treatment and children's progress.

The group consisted of four girls, who ranged in age from 6 to 9 years. Three girls were Hispanic, and the dominant language in their home was Spanish. In two of these homes, the parents were monolingual Spanish speaking. The other girl was African-American, and her family was monolingual English speaking. In the three Hispanic families, both parents were present, and in the black family, only the mother was present. Two of the girls were the eldest child in their families, and the other two were the youngest. One child had been referred for therapy a year prior to the start of the group. She had attended three individual sessions: however, her mother, as is the case with most parents of elective mute children, had not recognized that there was a problem because the child was speaking at home. All the children had normal developmental milestones for speech. Only one child, the youngest in the group, had undergone a trauma that might have had a possible effect on her speech—she was reported to have fallen and lacerated her neck at the age of 26 months. The child had been hospitalized for four days as a result, but the mother reported no change in speech patterns following this accident. As necessary, all the parents were seen in consultation with the therapists to discuss specific issues of their children's therapy. When needed, parental therapy was provided.

As mentioned previously, the four children had been referred to the therapists by their schools (four schools in the same school district). Comments from the referral sources indicated that none of the children had spoken in the classroom or the school since enrollment. All the children had psychological evaluations that indicated normal intelligence and no learning disabilities. Physical examinations confirmed that there was no organic reason for their absence of speech. Three of the children were receiving speech therapy at school following their evaluation by a speech pathologist.

The children had been seen for an individual evaluation with one or the other of the therapists and had begun individual treatment. In consultation, the two therapists decided to pool resources and provide group treatment because of the similarity in background, problems, and ages of the children.

The therapists prepared a broad outline of the group's structure and goals, which they explained to the parents and children in individual sessions. Having exhausted all available methods of eliciting speech from their children while in school, the parents welcomed the group treatment program as an innovative and viable alternative. Both parents and children agreed to participate for an unlimited number of sessions.

The program was not designed in detail in advance. Each session was individually planned based on the previous week's progress. Time was taken at the end of each group to inform parents of their child's progress and to plan individual goals for the next group.

The plan was to help the children examine their mutism in school in a therapeutic setting where they would be free to understand their anxieties, inhibitions, and the consequences of their behavior. A strong component of group treatment was a behavior modification technique used to elicit speech, both quantitatively and qualitatively. The therapists did not emphasize the number of utterances but rather that each child be at ease and capable of appropriate speech. Therefore, the therapists did not monitor the number of verbalizations but relied on their own clinical observations as well as the children's own and classroom teachers' evaluations in determining the need for further treatment. Desensitization techniques were also used to help the children, first to speak in the therapy room, then elsewhere in the building where treatment took place, and then in the surrounding community. In the first group meeting, goals for the children were set at a minimum level. The children were required to leave their parents in the waiting room and to accompany the therapists to a group room. Here, the initial goal was to have the children respond in nonverbal ways to the therapists. The first activity was to make an animal out of modeling clay.

Once the animal was made, the therapists asked the children to make the sound that the animal would make. They were given options in the way that they could respond verbally: (1) they could speak to the entire group, (2) they could speak to one member of the group, or (3) they could speak to either therapist. This gradual introduction of speech became an important component in the early stage of treatment.

Therapy continued with toy animals, storytelling, and tape recorders during the early sessions. Play materials such as paint, dolls, jump ropes, board games, and so forth were used to help the children express feelings. One of the rituals of the group was to say hello and good-bye to every group member in a verbal or nonverbal way. The nonverbal communication was much less anxiety provoking, and the children were able to touch, shake hands, or wave to comply with these goals.

The youngest client was very resistant to communicating with the therapists or other group members. It was decided that she would have individual sessions with one therapist prior to the beginning of the group so that verbal responses could be elicited on a one-to-one basis. By herself, the child responded much the same way that she did in the group; however, the therapist was able to elicit verbal responses. The therapist found that tickling the child was one way to lower defensiveness in the individual sessions. Achieving progress there, the child became more responsive in the group.

Focus in the group moved from fine motor play activities to those involving gross motor movement such as jumping rope. The introduction of these activities lowered anxiety in the group members, decreased feelings of incompetence and self-awareness, and provided them with additional ways to express themselves nonverbally. The therapists found that relaxation techniques and deep-breathing exercises facilitated speaking, and so they made these a regular part of the group ritual.

After the fourth group session, each child was required to respond in a verbal way at least once during the group meeting. The children began by whispering and thereafter moved on to a more appropriate tone and volume. The issue of the logical consequences of the children's behavior was also introduced; for example, they were told that if they would not speak in school, the results would be poor school performance, possible retention, and being socially stigmatized by peers. In discussing this, the children revealed that they were already the target of much hostility from school personnel.

By the end of the fifth session, all the children were able to respond verbally at least once during the group meeting. The children had moved from verbal responses of yes or no to one- or two-word sentences and then to longer sentences. At this time, the therapists began making contact with the children's schools to help their clients in the environment in which it was most difficult for them to speak. Treatment progressed from the group room to the outside environment. The therapists took the children to a park where they all played with water balloons. One type of interaction that seemed to produce a great deal of speech and satisfaction in the children was the formation of alliances between various group members and one or the other of the therapists. These alliances, which elicited speech from the children and helped them to develop a more trusting and genuine relationship with the therapists, represented a significant breakthrough. More nonverbal communication began, with children touching, pinching, or tickling the therapists. These activities were rewarded by positive reactions from the therapists, who also began shaping the children's behavior so that the touching and verbal responses were appropriate. The children's anger at their schools, their families, and even the therapists was explored. Subsequently, the therapists started to work with the children in other community settings, having them speak in a park, in a library, and in a restaurant. At this point, the children were ready to begin work on speaking at school.

With each child, work on speaking at school developed in a different way. One of the mothers enrolled her daughter in a new school at the end of the summer. When the child started school, the therapists consulted with the principal and the classroom teacher, advising them of the child's diagnosis and of approaches to successful resolution of the mutism. After the first week in school, the therapists learned that the child was talking there—the teacher expected the child to respond verbally and to discard her previous role as an elective mute. This complemented the therapists' treatment of the child and ensured continued success. When this development was discussed in the group, a second child requested to be transferred to a different school where she would not have to "play the role" of an elective mute.

Before transfer was explored, however, the therapists required that this 7-year-old child work on attaining the following goals: (1) talking in the group, (2) understanding consequences of her behavior, (3) improving self-esteem, (4) becoming assertive, (5) improving social skills, and (6) managing stress. Once the transfer became definite, the therapists instituted a desensitization program that included the following steps: (1) taking the child to the school when it was not in session, having her talk to the therapist, and walking around the school; (2) taking the child to the classroom, introducing her to the teacher and to the principal, and having her speak to both of them; (3) taking the child to the classroom and expecting her to talk with the students; and (4) leaving the child in the classroom for a full day to assess her verbal responses and coping skills.

This treatment plan proved to be successful. The final results were that all children were able to respond verbally in school. Furthermore, not only were the children able to speak in school, but also it was reported by the parents that the children had become much more spontaneous in speaking at home, were able to talk to others whereas they had been previously mute, and in addition, were able to improve peer relationships. In working with these children, it became evident that close cooperation with their schools was imperative. Unfortunately, cooperation between a school and a mental health center has many possible roadblocks. Overall, cooperation from the schools was forthcoming, but in one situation the child's teacher and the school were unwilling to assume their responsibility in the treatment plan (which then had to be postponed for a full year until the child transferred to another school). For this reason, prior to the treatment of an elective mute child, it is mandatory that the school become involved and consent to the treatment plan.

It is important to note that, in spite of inadequate space, lack of play equipment, and difficulty in coordinating the therapists' work with the schools' schedules, a 100 percent success rate was achieved when the treatment plan was followed. The therapists observed the children formally on a follow-up basis, and the children were succeeding in their school environment. Contact with the schools was made at three months, at six months, and at one year following the termination of treatment, at which times all four children were free of symptoms.

Although part of the treatment plan included transfer to a new school for each of the four children, this should not be interpreted as the primary resolution of the problem. Group psychotherapy was the essential ingredient to successful recovery. The transfer to another school secured the child's new role as a verbal member of her class and of society.

IMPLICATIONS

Treatment for elective mute children raises some questions that should be pursued. Are children who come from families in which another language is spoken at higher risk to be elective mutes? Was the fact that all referrals were members of a minority group significant? The two children most resistive to treatment were firstborns. Is this a prognosticator for treatment? These and other questions—leading to the need for further research on elective mutes and their treatment—are of interest to the therapeutic community.

Group treatment of elective mute children is a rare modality due to limited number of cases that a therapist is likely to encounter; however, should the opportunity present itself, this mode of therapy seems a natural and expedient way to treat children who have this devastating problem. Group treatment focuses on both nonverbal and verbal responses to the therapist and then is generalized to others within the community, thus helping the children to decrease their anxiety level, adopt productive and positive behavior patterns, and feel confident when using speech. The success rate is promising for those individuals who participate.

REFERENCES

American Psychiatric Association. (1980). *Diagnostic and Statistical Manual of Mental Disorders, Third Edition (DSM-III)*. Washington, DC: American Psychiatric Association.

Browne, E., Wilson, V., and Laybourne, P. C. (1963). Diagnosis and treatment of elective mutism in children. *Journal of the American Academy of Child Psychiatry* 2:605–617.

Chapin, A. B., and Corcoran, M. (1947). A program for the speech-inhibited child. *Journal of Speech and Hearing Disorders* 12:373–376.

Chethik, M. (1973). Amy: the intensive treatment of an elective mute. *Journal of the American Academy of Child Psychiatry* 12:482–498.

Halpern, W., Hammond, J., and Cohen, R. (1971). A therapeutic approach to speech phobia: elective mutism reexamined. *Journal of the American Academy of Child Psychiatry* 10:94–97.

Landgarten, H. B. (1981). *Clinical Art Therapy*. New York: Brunner/Mazel.

Mora, G., Devault, S., and Schopler, E. (1962). Dynamics and psychotherapy of identical twins with elective mutism. *Journal of Child Psychology and Psychiatry* 3:41–52.

Morris, J. V. (1953). Cases of elective mutism. *American Journal of Mental Deficiency* 57:661–668.

Nolan, J., and Pence, C. (1970). Operant conditioning principles in the treatment of a selectively mute child. *Journal of Consulting Clinical Psychology* 35:265–268.

Parker, E. B., Olsen, T. F., and Throckmorton, M. C. (1960). Social casework with elementary school children who do not talk in school. *Social Work* 5:64–70.

Reid, J. B., et al. (1967). A marathon behavior modification of a
    selectively mute child. *Journal of Child Psychology and Psychiatry*
    8:27–30.
Straughan, J. H., Potter, W. K., Jr., and Hamilton, S. H. (1965). The
    behavioral treatment of an elective mute. *Journal of Child Psy-
    chology and Psychiatry* 6:125–130.
Weinberger, G., Stander, R. J., and Stearns, R. P. (1967). Therapeu-
    tic strategies with school phobics. *American Journal of
    Orthopsychiatry* 37:64–70.

14

SIBLING GROUP PLAY THERAPY: AN EFFECTIVE ALTERNATIVE WITH AN ELECTIVE MUTE CHILD

Karen Barlow, JoAnna Strother, and Garry Landreth

BROWN AND LLOYD (cited in Kolvin and Fundudis 1981) reported that for every 1,000 children, there may be as many as 7.2 who do not speak at school at the age of 5. Kolvin and Fundudis (1981) defined this phenomenon, *elective mutism*, as "a strange condition where talking is confined to a familiar situation and a small group of intimates" (p. 219). They further reported that parents of elective mute children observed normal speech development when the children began to talk, but as they were placed in more social situations, shyness became prevalent.

ELECTIVE MUTISM AND ENURESIS

In this chapter we present the case study of Amy, a 5-year old elective mute, who was referred to the Pupil Appraisal Center (PAC) on the North Texas State University campus. Her mother referred her to the center because she was concerned about Amy's refusal to talk at school or in any situation away from the home. Amy also exhibited excessive shyness and suffered from enuresis, nighttime bed-wetting. Amy was the middle child in her nuclear family. She had two brothers. She seemed especially close to and dependent on her mother, which is common among elective mute children (Kolvin and Fundudis 1981).

Her mother initiated the process of play therapy and was the parent who followed through during the entire treatment period. Amy's father was never involved, but he was reported to be cooperative in the process at home. When counseling children, it is ideal for counselors to have both parents involved and informed. This case, however, demonstrates that play therapy can have positive results even though both parents are not involved in the parent consultation process.

In addition to being concerned with the elective mutism, Amy's mother also reported a concern over Amy's nighttime bed-wetting. Amy's brothers also suffered from this condition. In a study of twenty-four elective mute children, Kolvin and Fundudis (1981) reported a significantly high level of enuresis among the participants. They also found that these children had a higher ratio of behavioral problems, suffered from excessive shyness, exhibited more immaturity (especially in speech development), that more girls than boys were elective mutes, and that elective mutism proved to be rather intractible. The American Psychiatric Association (1980), in *The Diagnostic and Statistical Manual of Mental Disorders*, has also described elective mute children as suffering from excessive shyness, social isolation, behavioral difficulties, and, possibly, enuresis.

BEHAVIORS EXHIBITED

Amy's behavior and development paralleled that of children in the Kolvin and Fundudis (1981) study. According to Amy's teacher, she did seem to be developmentally behind and still suffered from enuresis at age 5. She was extremely shy and, according to her mother and teachers, exhibited some behaviors that were not normal for a child of her age. There were no distinguishable clues to the events that led to Amy's elective mutism. In their review of the literature, Kolvin and Fundudis found no specific or conclusive causes for elective mutism.

Amy did not speak one word during the first five months she was enrolled in the early childhood program at her school. She passed all the nonverbal items at the appropriate age level on an early childhood screening test and was put in a special education transition class. Amy's teachers observed her to be a passive little girl, who sat and observed activity around her. Her social skills were virtually nonexistent. She did not play with groups of children, but preferred to play alone or with an adult. When a new, quiet girl took a special interest in her, Amy did accept her. Initially the new girl talked to Amy, but later she just followed Amy's gesturing. As the school year progressed, Amy became more active and her facial expressions became more animated. She even smiled and laughed occasionally.

On the playground, Amy would linger on the playground and trail her classmates. She did not interact with the other children. When the teacher would take her hand to lead her to the sandbox or swings, Amy would pull away.

Amy displayed some additional unusual behaviors. She grasped the teacher aide's neck with her hands in a strong hold, smiling while she did it. She repeatedly stabbed the playhouse doll with a fork. She would wet her pants if the teachers forgot to ask her if she needed to go to the bathroom, although she had been told that she could go to the bathroom anytime.

Her mother reported that Amy did not show pain. She once sat in a tub of scalding water and just looked at her grandmother blankly when she asked Amy why she was still in the water. Amy had her pierced earrings pulled through her ears while playing and did not complain to the teacher, although her ears were bleeding. She fell in the gymnasium at school, which caused her mouth to bleed, and when the teacher asked her if it hurt, she shook her head from side to side. She did not show excitement or happiness on field trips or party days.

TEACHERS' EFFORTS

Amy's teachers used several techniques to elicit some type of verbal response. She was accepted as a nonverbal participant. On other occasions she was ignored when she would not respond verbally. When this failed, she was required to sit in a "time out" chair if she did not speak, but Amy seemed to take pleasure in sitting in the chair. According to her teacher, she was as sassy as anyone could be without saying a word. She did respond to being touched and on several occasions initiated sitting on the teacher's lap, following the lead of other children in the class. Amy was described by her teachers as passive, resistant, voluntarily nonverbal, occasionally hostile, compulsive and controlling, and emotionally unexpressive, as well as accepting of some people, responsive to affection, and willing to copy other children's behavior.

PLAY THERAPY

For a child exhibiting elected mutism, it is imperative that therapeutic communication be based on a means of expression with which the child feels comfortable. The counselor who relies exclusively on verbal means of communication with such children is often defeated in efforts to establish an effective relationship. The elective mute child easily controls the interaction with silence, thus also controlling development of the relationship with the counselor. Efforts to entice, encourage, cajole, or trick such children into a verbal exchange typically result in continued silence and a frustrated counselor.

The elective mute child has discovered from previous experiences what adults want—verbalization—and how to easily thwart their efforts by resisting through silence. Therefore, because play is the natural medium of self-expression for children, play therapy was selected as the preferred therapeutic approach with Amy. Her therapist believed Amy needed a therapeutic setting in which she could feel comfortable, a place where she could be in charge, within limits, of the relationship with an adult, and could communicate on her own terms without using words, as expected of her by other adults.

Regarding the value of play, Conn (1951) stated, "Every therapeutic play method is a form of learning process during which the child learns to accept and to utilize constructively that degree of personal responsibility and self-discipline necessary for effective self-expression and social living" (p. 753).

A SILENT BEGINNING

During the initial session in play therapy, Amy was totally nonverbal. She hid under the paint easel and gestured for 1 hour. The counselor responded with similar gestures and verbal comments, which she hoped would communicate understanding of her feelings. If the counselor remained motionless and silent for even a short time, Amy would look out from under the easel to make sure she still had the counselor's undivided attention. At the end of the session Amy readily emerged from under the easel.

Amy's cousin Susan accompanied her to the PAC for the second session. When Amy resisted returning to the playroom, the counselor invited Susan to come into the playroom too. Susan began talking as soon as the playroom door opened, and Amy returned to her hiding place under the easel. Susan played with many of the toys and after about 10 minutes, Amy joined her. They chatted back and forth and played contentedly for the hour. One would not have believed that there was anything unusual about Amy at this time.

This was such an unexpected turn of events that the counselor decided to add Amy's 9-year-old brother Ben to the third session to better understand the dynamics of Amy's interpersonal interactions. In this session, Susan and Ben played together and ignored Amy, who finally retreated into her hiding place under the easel. After the third session, Susan returned to her home in another town. The counselor had to decide whether to see Amy by herself or to include her older brother in the session. Amy also had a younger brother, Ned, who was very eager to come into the playroom.

SIBLING GROUP PLAY THERAPY

The question of placing siblings together in group play therapy has received little attention in the literature on play therapy. Ginott (1961) has been one of the few authors to even mention the issue of siblings; however, he has done so only in the context of recommending that children experiencing intense sibling rivalries be excluded from group play therapy. Consideration of placing siblings together is not mentioned.

The possibility of placing siblings together in group play therapy is often ruled out by requiring children selected for group play therapy to be the same age. According to Gazda (1978) and Ginott (1982), children in group play therapy should not differ in age by more than one year. Ginott did suggest that other considerations may take precedence over age, such as when aggressive children are placed in older age groups or immature children are placed in groups with children younger than themselves. Ginott further restricted the possibility of having siblings together in play therapy by recommending that school-age children be separated by sexes. We have found little need to separate children by sex until approximately the age of 8 or 9.

It seems reasonable to assume that the basic reasons for placing children in group play therapy may be equally as important for sibling group play therapy. If the presence of several children in the playroom helps to anchor the experience to the world of reality (Ginott 1961), this would seem to be even more true for siblings together in group play therapy. If, as Ginott (1961) proposed, children help each other assume responsibility in interpersonal relationships, the impact on siblings would be even more significant because of the opportunity to naturally and immediately extend those interactions with siblings outside the setting of group play therapy.

SEARCHING FOR THE RIGHT COMBINATION

In Amy's case, a combination of sibling play therapy, individual play therapy, and brief family consultation was found to be the most appropriate approach. When Amy played in the playroom with Ben, he was the responsible one—for himself and for Amy. She did not have to do anything; Ben talked and played for both of them. When Amy played in the playroom with Ned, she was the teacher and helper, although Ned was independent. When both boys came into the playroom, they played together and ignored Amy. When the children came into the room with their mother, they all tended to act out somewhat, but behaved with fairly equal exchanges.

When Amy played alone in the playroom, she remained shy, yet verbal. She would hide in her usual place under the easel for 10 or 15 minutes until she felt safe enough to emerge. Her play was often inappropriate, in the sense of periodic bursts of hostility or lengthy laughter or destructiveness. Modeling play behaviors that she had experienced with her brothers did generalize, however, to her individual play.

AMY'S NEED TO CONTROL

One theme continued for most of the play sessions. Amy wanted to be in total control and used silence to accomplish it. When the counselor continued to reflect her feelings verbally, she resented the loss of control. She repeatedly said, "Don't look at me. Don't talk to me." The counselor used a compromising approach on this issue. Amy was given control of "looks" and the counselor was given control of "talk." Amy seemed satisfied to have a well-defined area of control and was willing to let the counselor have one too. Gradually, Amy began to accept partial control in other areas. Ben and Amy divided the room into two parts. Each had to obtain verbal permission from the other to play in their respective control zones. Practicing, even in a structured way, the "give-and-take" that occurs naturally with many children seemed to give Amy the confidence she needed to develop her social skills, rather than to turn inward.

As Amy became more independent, Ben dropped his role as protector and responsible member of the family. He acted out to the extent that his mother had to discipline him publicly—a first in this family. During 15-minute family sessions after the sibling play therapy sessions, the counselor shared with the mother and children the changing pattern of communication between Ben and Amy. Ben gradually was able to let Amy be her own person and retain his significant position of being one of several responsible members of the family. The mother encouraged this shift in communication at home by giving Amy more responsibility and not allowing Ben to take over her tasks, even when he could do them better and faster. Ned also maintained a balanced independence, rather than adopting Amy's role of being helpless and in total control or Ben's role of being responsible and in total control. Amy began to express feelings more frequently. Raising her closed fist was her way of saying, "Don't come close to me," or "This will keep me safe when I have to walk close to you."

A DIFFERENT AMY

Amy's new confidence extended into the classroom. Talking, singing, and participating in class became fun for her. Her play sessions shifted to the school setting. She loved to be the teacher. When Amy would forget some mathematical fact or how to spell a new word she had learned, she would report what this word would be in Spanish. The counselor reflected the idea that sometimes only Amy would be able to tell what the word really meant. Amy's love of learning became evident in the safe environment of the playroom. She had initially concentrated on receiving information and not expressing it.

In later sessions Amy actively participated in expressing each new learning situation. The pace of Amy's progress was like a door bursting open. She even read a Christmas story over the loudspeaker at school. After nine months and thirty-six sessions of combining sibling play therapy, the final reward was Amy's assignment to a regular first-grade classroom in the spring of the year. As Amy became more verbal and more actively participated in her world, the enuresis began to occur less frequently.

SIGNIFICANCE OF SIBLING PLAY THERAPY

What was gained by having Amy's brothers in play therapy with her? As in family therapy, ideally, the focus shifts from intrapersonal to interpersonal patterns of communication. In this particular case, lack of verbal communication skills and underdeveloped social skills were paralyzing Amy's efforts to function in society beyond her immediate family.

It was obvious in sessions with Amy and her younger brother, Ned, that Amy had some basic social and communication skills. Observation of Ben and Amy in the playroom revealed that Ben had assumed responsibility for both himself and Amy. By helping Ben and Amy shift their ways of communicating, the counselor helped Amy to gain confidence to try a new way of entering the world of people instead of having someone take responsibility for her. Although individual play therapy might have eventually produced similar results, the sibling play therapy approach in this case seemed to bring faster results because the issues could be defined immediately, and work in sessions and at home could begin on the shift in the communication pattern.

We are not suggesting that sibling play therapy be used exclusively in every situation, or that it is the answer to cases in which the child has experienced trauma, but it can add a dimension to play therapy that previously has not been seriously considered. In fact, Amy definitely needed some time by herself to try out new behaviors learned in the setting that included her brothers, but the sibling setting served as a diagnostic tool for the counselor and as an intimate environment in which the client could model changed behaviors.

IMPLICATIONS FOR SCHOOL COUNSELORS

The infusion of group or sibling play therapy into a school counselor's developmental guidance program could have several valuable results:

1. In the case of an elective mute, play therapy could help the teacher and the child avoid a power struggle over talking. Play therapy is a nonverbal solution to a nonverbal problem.
2. Play therapy could provide a way to observe the child and the child's interactions with peers or siblings.
3. A play therapy experience could lead to more effective teacher-counselor consultation as a result of the counselor's relationship with the child.
4. The play therapy could help the child feel better about school as a result of a positive experience in the playroom.
5. The counselor would be better prepared to assist the parents as a result of the relationship with the child in play therapy.

SUMMARY

Kolvin and Fundudis (1981) stated that elective mutism is rather intractible. This chapter reported a case study in which sibling play therapy seems to have been a viable treatment for an elective mute child. The goals were to help Amy progress from an interpersonal communication pattern to an interpersonal pattern with others outside her family, to help her develop the courage to communicate verbally in school, and to help her family members deal with the anxiety related to Amy's unusual behavior.

Because elective mute children have a purpose for their behavior, verbal prodding by adults usually reaps few benefits. It only widens the gap between themselves and the child. The elective mute child has chosen not to communicate verbally with those outside the immediate family for reasons that may revolve around fear of social situations in which he or she is expected to interact verbally with others. It seems valuable, consequently, to provide an alternative for the child. With group and sibling play therapy, the school counselor can provide an atmosphere in which the child feels safe and where there is no pressure to talk. This type of therapy also provides the counselor an opportunity to observe the child with other children when communicating during play.

REFERENCES

American Psychiatric Association. (1980). *Diagnostic and Statistical Manual of Mental Disorders, Third Edition (DSM-III)*. Washington, DC: American Psychiatric Association.

Conn, J. H. (1951). Play interview therapy of castration fears. *American Journal of Orthopsychiatry* 25:747–754.

Gazda, G. M. (1978). *Group Counseling: A Developmental Approach*. Boston: Allyn & Bacon.

Ginott, H. G. (1961). *Group Psychotherapy with Children: The Theory and Practice of Play Therapy*. New York: McGraw-Hill.

——— (1982). Group play therapy with children. *In Play Therapy: Dynamics of the Process of Counseling with Children*, ed. G. L. Landreth, pp. 327–341. Springfield, IL: Charles C Thomas.

Kolvin, I., and Fundudis, T. (1981). Elective mute children: psychological development and background factors. *Journal of Child Psychology and Psychiatry and Allied Disciplines* 22:219–232.

PART VI

MULTIMODAL
TREATMENT

15

ELECTIVE MUTISM

Sander M. Weckstein, David D. Krohn,
and Harold L. Wright

DESCRIPTION OF DISORDER

Mutism as a presenting clinical symptom in children can be due to several different psychiatric and neurological disorders (Rutter 1977). Elective mutism represents a specific clinical syndrome initially described by Kussmaul in 1877 and named by Tramer in 1934. In this chapter we describe in detail a treatment approach developed at Hawthorn Center. Elective mutism is a relatively rare and particularly treatment-resistant condition in which children with normal verbal capabilities refuse to speak with people outside the family in most or all unfamiliar social situations, particularly on beginning school. Prevalence rates of 0.3 to 0.8 per 1,000 have been reported (Brown and Lloyd 1975, Fundudis et al. 1979). Although *DSM-IV* (American Psychiatric Association 1994) requires a one-month symptom duration to make the diagnosis, some authors have argued that this diagnosis should be made only in the presence of mutism of at least six months' duration (Kolvin and Fundudis 1981, Wilkins 1985)

due to the high rate of transient mutism found in children upon
entering school (Brown and Lloyd 1975).

Most authors have reported the electively mute child to be negativistic, oppositional, controlling, and manipulative (Browne et al.
1963, Hayden 1980, Kolvin and Fundudis 1981, Krohn et al. 1992,
Parker et al. 1960, Wergeland 1979, Wilkins 1985, Wright 1968). They
are also described as shy and anxious in public; however, they may
be either shy or outgoing around familiar people (Kolvin and
Fundudis 1981, Parker et al. 1960, Wright 1968).

The relationship between the mother and child is often described as symbiotic, with the mother overprotecting and overindulg-
ing the child (Browne et al. 1963, Hayden 1980, Parker et al. 1960,
Wilkins 1985, Wright 1968). Hayden (1980) reported her observation
that the mothers appeared jealous of the child's interactions with
others. The marital relationship is usually described as conflictual,
with the father often uninvolved, and it is hypothesized that this is
the reason the mother turns to the child (Browne et al. 1963, Parker
et al. 1960, Wergeland 1979). Nevertheless, the only two controlled
studies have not found family discord to be higher in these families
as compared to families of other emotionally disturbed children
(Kolvin and Fundudis 1981, Wilkins 1985). Some authors have commented on a general lack of family communication (Hayden 1980,
Parker et al. 1960). Several authors have noted a general family shyness, history of shyness in the parents, or elevated levels of anxiety
in the parents (Hayden 1980, Kolvin and Fundudis 1981, Parker et
al. 1960, Wergeland 1979, Wright 1968).

Six studies reporting treatment results for more than ten cases
are available in the literature. Browne and colleagues (1963), reporting ten cases, and Wergeland (1979), reporting eleven, described using
a primarily psychodynamic approach and found the treatment long
and difficult with a generally poor outcome. Parker and colleagues
(1960), using a treatment approach that involved individual therapy,
family work, and school consultation, reported that all twenty-seven
of the elective mutes treated in their sample spoke within two years
of beginning treatment. Their admission criteria, however, did not

control for length of mutism, and success was defined only as "some use of speech" in the classroom. Kolvin and Fundudis's (1981) study of twenty-four electively mute children described 46 percent showing marked to moderate improvement and 54 percent slight to no improvement. The duration of mutism and the treatment technique were not clearly described.

Wright's original (1968) report on nineteen patients found 79 percent to have an excellent or good outcome, whereas 21 percent had a fair to poor outcome (including one schizophrenic). A later additional study of twenty strictly diagnosed elective mutes using the Hawthorn Center approach found a similar high treatment success rate with eighteen (90 percent) having an excellent outcome and two (10 percent) a fair outcome (Krohn et al. 1992).

There are also no larger studies on behavioral therapy of elective mutism, although many of the more recent articles propose this approach (Wright et al. 1985). Behavioral therapy techniques to treat elective mutism are well described (Labbe and Williamson 1984, Sanok and Ascione 1979, Sanok and Striefels 1979). There has been very little written on possible pharmacological interventions in the treatment of elective mutism. One successful case report of the use of Prozac has been reported (Black and Uhde 1992).

DIFFERENTIAL DIAGNOSIS

There has been some disagreement in the field as to whether elective mutism is an anxiety disorder, a specific developmental delay, or part of an oppositional defiant disorder. Previous experience by the present authors suggests that elective mutism is a symptom that must be understood in the context of each individual case history. Any of a number of factors may predispose the child to developing mutism, but the syndrome of elective mutism represents a final common behavioral pathway that develops when mutism becomes entrenched because of the gratification (secondary gain) it brings the child. These children are often anxious when forced to speak, but their anxiety is not pervasive. They are not typically shy or anxious when playing or interacting in other ways, even when being observed, but appear more controlling and oppositional.

Many disorders can also coexist with or present in a manner similar to elective mutism. The evaluator must be cognizant of the nonspecific nature of mutism as a presenting symptom and use the presence or absence of other associated symptoms to rule out possible affective spectrum disorder, anxiety disorder (specifically posttraumatic stress disorder [PTSD] and social phobia), speech and language disorder, oppositional-defiant disorder, or psychoses. If the history is suggestive of a diagnosis of elective mutism, the child is nonverbal and does not participate, and other major psychiatric disorders do not appear to be present, a diagnosis of elective mutism can be made.

ASSESSMENT PROCEDURES

A thorough evaluation is the first part of the treatment process. This includes obtaining a complete social history of the child from parents or primary caregivers including the onset, duration, precipitants, and a detailed understanding of the presentation itself as it occurs in different settings (i.e., home, school, and community). A history of the previous interventions or treatments and their results needs to be obtained. In addition, a developmental and medical history should be taken with specific emphasis on possible early speech and language problems or significant physical traumas to the mouth or other areas. A detailed history of the child's motor, language, and social development should also be obtained.

A family history including information about family constellation, relationships, and how the child's mutism is perceived and reacted to by the family is extremely important. It is also useful to ask whether there is a history of elective mutism or use of selective speech in any family members. Information about the current and past stability of the marital relationship should also be obtained. Finally, questions about a family history of psychiatric illness including depression, anxiety disorders, psychosis, and other mental disabilities should be elicited. Observing the child in free play or the family and child interacting in the waiting room is often very useful.

The clinical interview of the child is one of the most important parts of the evaluation process. The interviewer must be extremely cognizant of the child's appearance, cooperativeness, relatedness, and ability to separate from specific family members. If the child is uncooperative and not verbally interactive (as elective mutes often are at first), the interviewer should obtain information nonetheless by attempting to use nonverbal communication through play or art. It is important from the first session to attempt to build a therapeutic alliance, by facilitating interaction between the child and interviewer.

How then can this child, who has been so firmly entrenched in his symptom of silence (a symptom that both controls others and keeps others at a distance) be approached? The child must be drawn into the evaluation and subsequent therapy through play, interpretation, and a pragmatic explanation of the need to give up the symptom so he can make friends and learn. The therapist must be creative in gaining the child's interest and participation. The use of puppets, magic tricks, drawing, playful nonverbal communication such as imitating the child's posture and stance, and supportive interpretation of his feelings can be very useful.

Psychological testing including assessing intellectual functioning, academic achievement, and relevant dynamics is often used as one part of a comprehensive evaluation. However, since when first seen these children are often nonverbal and refuse to participate, more formal psychological testing often must be postponed until later in treatment.

ESTABLISHING TREATMENT GOALS

Helping the child, school, and family extricate themselves from the child's mutism is the main focus of treatment. This usually requires individual therapy for the child, family therapy, and school consultation, initially on at least a weekly basis. The treatment approach can be broadly broken down into nine different stages, all of which must be accomplished for treatment to be successful. These stages should be seen as flexible and they often overlap. They are (1) explaining the proposed technique to the child, family, and school, and acquiring their support of the treatment approach; (2) establishing rapport with the child; (3) the child speaking in response to the setting of the first verbal expectation in a session; (4) generalizing verbal production within the therapy session; (5) continuing exploration of the symptoms and their meaning; (6) generalizing positive verbal and nonverbal behaviors in the school setting simultaneous with generalizing in the community through parental involvement; (7) continuing reinforcement of the child's verbal activities and facilitating of an increased sense of mastery; (8) treating related problems of elective mutism once the symptom remits; and (9) gradually terminating treatment.

ROLE OF THE THERAPIST

The role of the therapist in this approach is a difficult one involving a combination of emphatic striving to form an alliance with the child and firm limit setting. It is important to be cognizant of the therapist's possible reactions concerning this approach to the treatment of elective mutism. When faced with treating one of these nonverbal children who can be seen as pathetic, controlling, oppositional, frustrating, overwhelming, anxious awe-inspiring, depressed, or angry, the therapist must be aware of his evoked feelings. These may run the gamut from anger to helplessness. The therapist must use his own feelings as an ally to help him interpret to the child what it must feel like to be silent, be it frightened or angry, controlling or passive. This helps the child realize that someone is trying to understand his predicament and will do something to help. The therapist must be comfortable with the feelings the child evokes in him as he sets a firm, but appropriate, limit while the child may be crying, whining, standing rigidly in the corner, or trying to escape. Those who come from a more analytic or nonstructured therapeutic background may be uncomfortable with this technique. It has been our experience at Hawthorn Center, using this approach with numerous children, that it is usually effective. This treatment technique does not cause the symptoms of elective mutism to be replaced by others, and will not be harmful to the child when it is carried out by an empathetic therapist with a clear understanding of the symptom, treatment technique, and child development. In fact, the children report and manifest much relief when their symptom is removed. As we previously mentioned, this technique is designed to facilitate ego growth and mastery for those children who are developmentally arrested by their symptom and cannot find a way to extricate themselves from their situation.

TREATMENT STRATEGIES

The first stage of treatment consists of explaining the proposed techniques to the family and actively acquiring the family's assistance in such a way that the family is not threatened. It is further necessary to have the family's assistance in not condoning the child's silence. The therapist's role in this phase of treatment is supportive and psychoeducational. Elective mutism is explained as an extremely detrimental symptom that can seriously impede normal development and, therefore, requires prompt intervention so the child can successfully make friends, progress appropriately in school, and not feel badly about himself because he cannot do what other children are doing. This phase of treatment is usually completed within the first two sessions.

Once the family gives support for the treatment, the therapist must attempt to establish rapport with the child by demonstrating concern and understanding of the child's emotional distress and need for his symptom as well as show the child the importance of giving up his symptom. This is crucial to the ultimate success of the treatment. It is this approach, which combines an insistence that the child give up his silence with the message that the therapist will stick with the child, that provides the basis for sustained progress in treatment.

Each therapist has his own style of relating to the child, but this needs to be done in a fairly short period of time over the first two or three sessions with the child. Though one might be tempted to continue this phase of the treatment for a much longer period of time, it is important to let the child know that the therapist (unlike previous adults and children) will not be controlled by the child's symptom and accept continued silence, but will instead help the child to extricate him or herself.

After rapport has been established, the therapist supportively but firmly conveys to the child that he will be expected to talk in the near future. The child is told that while the therapist understands talking to people outside of the family is difficult, it is something that is necessary. Further, the child is told that there will come a time in the near future (the next one to two sessions) at which the child will be expected to say at least one word before leaving the session. The therapist directly states to the child that he will stay with the child as long as is necessary to accomplish this task. The idea that once he talks he will feel better about himself, that the first few words are the hardest, as well as the fact that it will be more fun for him when he can talk and play like other children, is emphatically explained and repeatedly highlighted to the child.

To accomplish the step of setting the first verbal expectation the therapist must schedule a day when he can spend enough time with the child to accomplish the first verbal task of saying at least one word to the therapist. In the majority of cases the session where the verbal expectation is set should occur by the third or fourth session with the child. The therapist should anticipate spending an extended period of time with the child and plan to have food and paperwork available and the resolve to carry through to the goal. Throughout the session the therapist periodically discusses the expectation that in order to end the session the child must say at least one word. The therapist alternates between being supportive, interpreting the child's feelings, attempting to engage the child in play, and seemingly ignoring the child at times. The times when the therapist seemingly ignores the child serve the purpose of allowing the child to go at his own pace, as well as clearly conveying to the child that the therapist will maintain a firm limit and not be controlled by the mutism.

After the child is verbal, the child is praised for his ability to master the situation, is told that he will continue to feel better about himself as he talks more, and is told he will be expected to be increasingly verbal at the next session. Then the child is taken back to his family, who have been instructed to praise the child's accomplishment.

The next stage of treatment consists of attempting to increase the child's verbalizations within the therapy framework while continuing to build a therapeutic alliance. This should be done in such a way that it is enjoyable for the child. It is often helpful to have the child bring in familiar objects, toys, or pictures. The child is encouraged to continue to be verbal by making a verbal response necessary for any activity that the child chooses. In some children this is not necessary, as they talk to the therapist in session fairly normally after they have completed the first verbal hurdle. Further, many children enjoy reading, naming colors or body parts, or talking about pictures that they have brought. We have found it important at this point to ask the child to do only things that he is capable of doing and has done before with family members. As stated before, the sense of mastery and enhancement of self-esteem that the child receives by being increasingly verbal in these ways with a therapist is tremendously reinforcing to the continued use of speech. Nevertheless, the therapist should use praise as well as other tangible reinforcers as needed.

The next phase consists of further exploration of the symptom by using play therapy techniques to help the child gain insight into his fears, fantasies, and concerns. The specific areas that need to be addressed in therapy vary significantly from child to child depending on what treatment discloses as the conflicts that led the child to develop the symptom of elective mutism. Often issues of anger, low self-esteem, passive aggressiveness, and oppositional behavior arise and are dealt with as the treatment continues. As the symptom remits, the child's developmental growth continues and tends to proceed along appropriate developmental lines. The child is happier, feels better about himself, and his anxiety and feelings of inferiority are replaced by feelings of mastery and a sense of self-worth.

The next phase of therapy involves generalization of verbal and nonverbal mastery to the school setting. This phase is begun after a strong therapeutic alliance has been formed and the child is comfortably speaking with the therapist. This can usually be accomplished between two weeks and three months from beginning therapy.

This phase requires the teacher's time and effort and, thus, a good working relationship with the teacher and the school is necessary for success. Shortly after treatment begins, it is important to contact, with parental approval, the child's principal, teacher, and school social worker to develop a dialogue and working relationship with the school staff who will be involved with the child's treatment. Often the school is the source of the referral and will contact the therapist with questions after the initial evaluation. It is helpful to briefly explain your treatment plan to those involved and then suggest to them that in the near future you will be contacting them to enlist their aid in the transfer of the child's verbal ability from the therapy to the school setting.

In preparing the child for this next step, the therapist must focus on the child's newfound verbal industry and self-mastery and side with the child's desire to "talk" and "be like other kids" or "show how smart he is." Further, the child's previous verbal accomplishments in therapy are highlighted and praised. The child's anxieties should be explored and addressed by suggesting that after the child becomes verbal in the school setting, he will feel better about himself, just as he does now in therapy. Then, a specific verbal task should be selected, practiced, and mastered. This may include reading a particular story or naming particular colors or body parts. This task should be repeatedly practiced in the sessions with much positive reinforcement.

Desensitization through role-playing and imagining what it

might be like to talk in the school setting can also be very helpful for the child. If the child's ambivalence is expressed through oppositional behavior and refusal, it should be addressed. A pragmatic explanation of why speaking is important, for example, "If you don't speak, the teacher cannot know how smart you are," can be given to the child. At the same time, positive reinforcers of tangible gifts, "I have a secret, special surprise waiting for you when you talk," the family's pride in the child's verbal accomplishments, and the fact that he will feel better about himself can be used.

The next step is to set a day on which the child is expected to speak in school. This is done with the collaboration of school personnel, and the specific details of the process are explained so that the teacher and other staff are able to participate fully.

The child is first given the opportunity to perform the preselected verbal task alone with the teacher. If this is unsuccessful after a few tries, the therapist should consider going to the school to help facilitate the generalization of verbal behaviors to the teacher.

After the child has begun speaking to the teacher alone, the teacher should continue to meet with the child individually on a daily basis for a period of time. The therapist then helps the teacher to generalize the child's verbal behaviors to the rest of the class, using both positive and negative reinforcement. However, as time goes on the reinforcement of being able to speak again, to socialize with peers and teachers, and the rewards of self-mastery should take the place of tangible rewards. Finally, after the child is comfortable with the selected teacher, that teacher may further generalize the child's verbal abilities in school to other teachers using the above described techniques.

Once the child is comfortable in being verbal in the therapy setting and is working on being verbal in the school setting, it is time to further the generalization of the child's verbal behavior in the community through the family. It is important at this time to attempt to explore and understand the child's symptom choice and the dynamics behind it in the family setting. Often, with elective mutism, there is some overenmeshment of the family. In addition, family members may be perpetuating the symptom. Therapeutic work with the family is directed at helping them recognize and acknowledge their symptom-perpetuating behaviors, thus developing a collective observing ego. Further, it is often important to counsel parents on techniques of firm and appropriate limit setting.

At this phase in the treatment a reassessment is indicated. One should determine whether additional interventions are needed such as intensive family therapy or referral of other family members for individual treatment, or whether the treatment of the child and limited family work is sufficient to deal with the specific problems. Further, during this part of therapy, the therapist should continue to explore the child's symptom in individual therapy. He should also reinforce the child's gains, his industry, and his self-mastery through play and verbal means.

DEALING WITH COMMON OBSTACLES TO SUCCESSFUL TREATMENT

One of the common challenges to the successful treatment of elective mutism is maintaining an alliance with the family throughout the treatment. The therapist should anticipate the possibility of a family stopping treatment if the child appears unhappy or angry, because these parents have usually been controlled by the child previously. This issue should be anticipated and addressed by explaining to the parents that during the treatment there may well be times when the child seems unhappy and angry and will not want to come to the sessions. Their child may direct his anger at them in such a way as to make them feel guilty or uncomfortable, but it is important to continue treatment, even if they are uncomfortable with this technique. Parents are told that other parents have felt this way in the past, but with continued treatment, their children improved. It is reiterated that they are the most important people in their child's life and their continued participation in the treatment is paramount. Often families may be noncompliant with treatment suggestions and this must be gently pointed out as evidence of their ambivalence and the issue addressed. Further, introducing techniques of using concrete props such as star charts, lists, or worksheets can be useful. It is important to involve all family members in treatment. If one or another parent is more distant (often the father in elective mute families), he or she should be encouraged to join in the treatment.

We have found that some mothers of elective mutes encourage, convertly or overtly, their child's mutism because of their need to keep the child dependent, often because of their own unresolved dependency needs or dissatisfaction in the marriage (Krohn et al. 1992). This must be evaluated and approached in a sensitive manner. It is important to highlight the child's gains to the family members as well as to give the family members much of the credit for these gains while at the same time discussing the family members' ambivalence about the child's increasing mastery and decreased dependence.

The most difficult part of this treatment (for the therapist as much or more than the child) is the session in which the verbal expectation is set. Children with elective mutism have often had years of practice in bringing family members, teachers, principals, and often therapists to their knees over the issues of mutism. The child's own ambivalence about this symptom and the negative effect it has on a child's development must always be remembered.

It is very important not to allow the child to leave the session in which the limit is set without talking unless both the child and the therapist are both physically and emotionally exhausted. At times, in very difficult cases, it has been useful to tell the child that it is not fair to keep his mother or family waiting any longer. He is told that the family will be sent home and will return later in the day when the child is verbal. This serves to raise the child's anxiety and show that the family will no longer be controlled by the child's mutism. If the child is verbal in any manner (whiny or whispered words), the therapist may choose to accept and reinforce this response with the understanding that next time it must be more audible, or continue to wait for a more audible response.

RELAPSE PREVENTION

Children treated with the Hawthorn Center approach have had a very low rate of relapse. This is in large part due to the work done with the families of the children. The families' commitment to encouraging and reinforcing their child's verbal participation in all settings by establishing appropriate and firm limits when needed is crucial to treatment and to prevention of relapse. During the active phase of the treatment, the families work through the conflicts and understand the dynamics of the role that they usually have played in their child's mutism. The understanding and confidence they have gained and the commitment they have to their child's continued healthy growth and development, which they come to realize requires appropriate speech, allows them to follow through with the treatment plan as described and not fall back into the pattern of giving in to their child's mutism. Along with this, the understanding and commitment of school personnel in requiring the child's verbal participation in the school setting is important. Finally, the child's newfound abilities of being able to speak freely and to socialize with family, peers, and others is tremendously reinforcing. As the child's verbal abilities increase, the child develops an increased sense of mastery over himself and the world around him. This sense of mastery serves to further perpetuate the child's continued growth.

TERMINATION

When the child is functioning at a developmentally appropriate level and his symptoms have resolved, it is time for a gradual termination of treatment. The time between the child's appointments is slowly increased in length, depending on the child's needs, over a two- to six-month period of time. A gradual termination allows the child to slowly break the strong bond with the therapist that often develops during the treatment. The issues of loss precipitated by the planned termination of therapy must be approached and worked through before treatment can be successfully ended. The child should be told that he may return to therapy even after termination if ever he feels the need.

During the termination phase, the child may show some regression, such as a recurrence of controlling behaviors. Working with the family or school to set appropriate limits and discussing feelings and fears about control with the child will usually resolve these behaviors.

CASE ILLUSTRATION (TYPICAL TREATMENT)

DESCRIPTION AND HISTORY

Jonathan was a 7-year-old first grader when initially seen. He had not spoken for the first four months of first grade, had spoken only a few words in the first month of kindergarten before refusing to speak, and had not spoken in day care, which he attended for a year prior to attending kindergarten. His mother said that she was surprised when he began not speaking in school as he was quite animated and outgoing at home and with the family. She did state that he was extremely reluctant to talk in public but that she had thought that this was normal for his age. She said that she was initially not bothered by his mutism and was seeking the evaluation at the teacher's request. Jonathan was described as having no other emotional or behavioral difficulties but as being a somewhat strong-willed and stubborn child.

Jonathan's development and medical history were unremarkable. Language milestones were recalled as being normal. Jonathan lived at home with his mother and an older brother. Jonathan's father had left the family somewhat suddenly when Jonathan was 3 years of age. He had little contact with the family after leaving the home.

Jonathan's family history was also unremarkable. There was no family history of mental illness. Jonathan's mother recalled that she herself had been somewhat quiet in school and that it was hard for her to speak in the early grades.

SYNOPSIS OF THERAPY SESSIONS

When seen for the initial evaluation, Jonathan refused to speak to the evaluator, although he was observed to speak quietly with his mother in the waiting room. The evaluator was, however, able to initiate animated and interactive play using puppets and allowing him to shoot basketball in the room. His play was very logical and coherent and he appropriately followed the nonverbal social cues of the examiner. The results of Jonathan's evaluation were discussed with his mother.

> Therapist: After going over the information you presented to us and having a chance to spend some time with Jonathan, I feel Jonathan has a problem called elective mutism.
>
> Mother: That's what the teacher said when she said I should call you, but I still don't understand what elective mutism is.
>
> Therapist: Elective mutism is a problem in which a child with normal speech abilities refuses to speak with people outside of the family in most or all unfamiliar situations. So Jonathan is able to speak normally, but he's fallen into a pattern of not talking that needs to stop.
>
> Mother: Is it really anything we have to worry about?
>
> Therapist: It is a serious problem, but fortunately it can be successfully treated. All children's intellectual, social, and emotional growth in the early years is largely based on their ability to verbally interact with other children and adults at home, school, and in the community. Though this can be accomplished to a certain extent by gestures, Jonathan's refusal to speak puts him at a tremendous disadvantage. He will have, and is already having, a very difficult time making and keeping friends, as well as learning and interacting in a normal manner at school. These things will likely lead to him feeling badly about himself as he sees he is not able to do what the other children are doing.

Mother: Why does Jonathan have this problem? Is it my fault?

Therapist: No, it's not a matter of fault. Kids fall into the pattern of being silent for many reasons. Once they do, however, they often get lots of attention for their silence as other people talk and do things for them. That's an easy pattern for families and parents to fall into, as it is natural to want to do anything to help your child or make them feel more comfortable. I think Jonathan and you have gone through a lot, and there are many positive things about Jonathan. I don't know all the reasons Jonathan stopped talking, and we probably won't know for a while, but we need to get Jonathan back on track talking as quickly as possible.

Mother: You know, I think I have gotten into the habit of talking for Jonathan and doing things for him too. I was only trying to help. So now what? How can we help my son?

Therapist: Fortunately, as I said before, elective mutism is a very treatable problem and we had the chance to successfully treat many children with elective mutism here at Hawthorn Center.

The treatment technique was described to Jonathan's mother. When told of the detrimental effect of not speaking, she described how she had lately been worried as he was not making friends and that she had observed him in school being somewhat lonely and isolated. She was in agreement with the treatment plan. Jonathan was told at the evaluation that at the next session he would be expected to speak.

An appointment was then scheduled for the next week. The therapist cleared his schedule of patients in the morning and made prior arrangements to possibly cancel meetings that were planned for the afternoon. Jonathan came readily to the therapist's office and when asked how he was doing responded, "Fine," while walking back to the office. Upon entering the office he stood in a corner and was more reticent than when previously seen. When asked another question after entering the office, he refused to speak. After a few minutes, he pointed at the basketball and indicated nonverbally that he wanted to again shoot baskets. As a good rapport was felt to have been established during the evaluation and as Jonathan had spoken coming back to the office, the therapist made the decision to require Jonathan to name the toy with which he wished to play. After approximately thirty seconds Jonathan pointed to the basketball and said, "Basketball." Following this session he was taken back to the waiting room after being given much praise by the therapist. His mother also praised him and announced that he would be taken for ice cream for having spoken during the session.

In the first half of the next session Jonathan spoke very softly and offered very little speech other than naming the toy with which he wished to play. During the second half of session he was required to speak progressively louder the word *basketball* to have it rebounded for him. By the end of the session he was yelling the word *basketball* and appeared to enjoy this.

At the next session, after initially being required to get to the point of yelling the word *basketball*, he was told that he would have to say progressively one more word in order to have the basketball rebounded for him. By the end of the session he was saying strings of twenty-two words.

The following session the same limit was again imposed but by the end of the session, as he ran out of things to name, Jonathan stated that he would rather just talk, and the guideline was set that he had to say a sentence before the ball would be rebounded. The therapist and Jonathan also spoke during that and the next session about what would be the easiest thing for him to say in the classroom. He felt that answering to the attendance roll call would probably be the easiest. This was practiced by having both the therapist and Jonathan practice answering, using a wide range of voices, volumes, and tones. His teacher was called and it was arranged that at a particular roll call he would be expected to answer. Jonathan was able to do this approximately one month after the first limit-setting session. On the same day as answering attendance, he also read a sentence aloud to the class when it was his turn to read without any additional prompting by the teacher. In subsequent sessions we continued to work on reading and increasing his verbal fluency.

In addition to the individual work with Jonathan, Jonathan's mother was seen on a biweekly basis. Four weeks into the treatment she spontaneously stated that she had been wondering if she had given Jonathan a covert message not to speak to others outside of the home because of her own difficulties in handling the abandonment by her husband. She also described how she felt she may have been supporting Jonathan becoming too dependent on her because of her own loneliness.

Six weeks into treatment she stated she had begun on her own to require Jonathan to speak in the community, as she felt he was ready. She described that beginning about a week after Jonathan spoke in the therapy session, they went out to dinner as a family. She told Jonathan prior to going out that he would have to order his own dinner. When he refused to speak in the restaurant, he did not receive dinner. The family afterward went out for ice cream and the same condition was set for Jonathan and she described how Jonathan had no difficulty in ordering ice cream. Since that time he had been able to order in restaurants and had also been able to speak with a librarian at the public library.

By three months after beginning treatment, Jonathan was speaking appropriately in the home, school, and community. His mother indicated that she had resumed dating again and she had sought her own individual therapy to address her difficulties with trust. A planned tapered termination was then instituted in which Jonathan came every two weeks for two sessions, then a month later, and then two months later. Jonathan continued to speak appropriately in all settings. At the final session, when asked, he stated that he did not remember why he had refused to speak in school and described feeling much happier now that he could. He proudly stated that he had made a number of new friends both in school and in his neighborhood.

COMMENTS

Jonathan represents a fairly typical treatment course for elective mutism using this technique. With the therapist's facilitation and appropriate limit setting the child usually is verbal the first session following the explanation of the expectation. While it was somewhat unusual in that he spoke coming back to the therapy room, most children are usually verbal after fifteen minutes to one hour in the session where the verbal expectation is set. After the child is over the first verbal hurdle, increasing speech within each session becomes progressively easier. In most elective mutes the feelings of increased mastery that occur as each fearful hurdle is overcome are tremendously reinforcing and speech becomes generalized in most settings with decreasing difficulty.

CASE ILLUSTRATION (OVERCOMING OBSTACLES)

DESCRIPTION AND HISTORY

Mark Wilson (a pseudonym) was a 6½-year-old boy who was seven months into first grade when he came to Hawthorn Center for evaluation. Mark's parents related to us that Mark had always had problems talking and "never really talked a lot" and "only to certain people."

The Wilsons told us that in kindergarten Mark initially refused to talk, but in the middle of the year did say single words to the teacher on a few occasions in response to being told by the teacher that he had to speak before he would be allowed to leave school. He returned to being totally mute for the last three months of kindergarten as the teacher did not follow through with her limit setting. In first grade, Mark returned to being totally mute in school. In both kindergarten and first grade, Mark never talked to others, participated spontaneously, ate in school, or used the bathroom. He would often stand in the corner refusing to participate.

The Wilsons downplayed the seriousness of Mark's problems,

telling us that they came to Hawthorn Center primarily because the school social worker "thought it would be helpful." The Wilsons further described Mark as a perfectionistic, strong-willed, and moody child. When angry, he would often respond by screaming, kicking, throwing a temper tantrum, or refusing to talk. In the community, Mark was described as a shy, withdrawn, clingy child who would not talk with anyone outside a few select people.

Mark's developmental milestones were described as unremarkable other than Mrs. Wilson stating that Mark was very resistant to toilet training until approximately 3½ years of age, but "when he decided to do it, it was no problem." Mark's past medical and developmental histories were essentially unremarkable.

Mark was in a dynamic insight-oriented therapy for approximately six months before coming to Hawthorn Center. During that period of time, Mark never talked to his therapist.

On first observing the Wilson family in the waiting room, Mark and Mrs. Wilson were noted to be sitting extremely close to one another with Mrs. Wilson's arm encircling him. Mr. Wilson was sitting off to the side.

In the first interview, Mark presented as a small boy who stood rigidly in the corner, with downcast eyes, whimpering, and remaining a silent nonparticipant throughout the interview. Mark further refused to participate in psychological testing that day and in that setting also stood rigidly in the corner unresponsive to attempts to engage him in the testing process.

SYNOPSIS OF THERAPY SESSIONS

The treatment technique was explained to the Wilsons, including the fact that after the child becomes comfortable with his therapist and rapport has developed, the therapist would make a morning appointment for the child and set aside the day with the expectation that the child say at least one word in the therapy session. The Wilsons were informed that Mark would be told that he would not be allowed to leave until he spoke. The Wilsons expressed their concern that this might in some way hurt Mark. They said, "The

other therapist said she could get Mark to talk, but if she forced him
it would hurt him." This issue was explored in depth and the Wilsons
were assured that this technique had been used very successfully with
many children over a number of years and had not been found to
be harmful. In addition, they were told it helps children to feel better about themselves when used by a person who is sensitive to the
child's feelings and who understands elective mutism. It was further
explained that, for treatment to be successful, family support is imperative, for it is the family and not the therapist who would ulti-
mately make the difference. The Wilsons expressed some skepticism
but agreed to the treatment.

Mark's reaction to being told he must say at least one word
before leaving the next session was a controlled, rigid, pitiful cry.
Nonetheless, an appointment was set with the Wilsons and the therapist cleared his schedule for the day. The Wilsons were told to bring
Mark in the morning and expect to spend a portion or all of the
day at Hawthorn Center.

Mr. and Mrs. Wilson arrived as scheduled with Mark at 8:00
A.M. on the day of the appointment. Mark was tearful and rigid and
refused to go with the therapist. Mr. Wilson picked Mark up in a
warm but firm manner (with the therapist's prompting) and carried
him to the therapist's office. He then succeeded in disentangling
himself from Mark and left. Mark stood rigidly in the corner, whimpering. The therapist asked Mark why he was crying but Mark did
not answer. The therapist told Mark that he knew it was scary for
him to be in the therapist's office and he was probably feeling angry
and frightened about talking, but nonetheless, today was the day
and the therapist would be willing to stay all day with him if needed
for Mark to talk.

The therapist initially tried to engage Mark by asking him if
he might want to talk now and tell the therapist with which game
or toy he wanted to play. Mark was silent. The therapist got out
some animal figures and played with them near Mark in an attempt
to involve him, but he would not participate. Playfully, the therapist made a small dog figure crawl up Mark's leg and his stomach to

his shoulder and finally to talk to Mark. Mark stood with his arms rigidly at his sides and tried to push the figure away with his body but would not use his hands to accomplish this task. The therapist created a voice for the dog figure, which told Mark that it was scared and then ran down Mark's body and hid in Mark's sock. This effort produced a small smile, which he quickly tried to hide. Then the dog figure (with some of his animal friends) attempted to get Mark to play with the animals or talk to them. Mark remained silent. An interpretation of how scary it must be to have to be the boss all the time was made to Mark through the dog figure.

The therapist told Mark that he had helped many other children with this problem and that Mark would feel better about himself after talking. The therapist then told Mark that if he wanted to do anything or play anything, he had but to ask, but if not, the therapist would then go and work on some paperwork at his desk. However, Mark would not be allowed to go home until he said at least one word. This statement caused Mark to cry once again.

This approach, which involved alternating between being supportive, clarifying feelings, encouraging Mark to participate, setting firm limits, and at times pretending to ignore Mark and do paperwork, continued for approximately four hours. Lunch was eaten in the room. Food and drink for Mark were placed on a table, but Mark stood rigidly in the corner, whimpering. Finally, much to the therapist's relief, Mark began quietly, with a closed mouth, to attempt to whine something. The therapist reacted to this by coming over to Mark to ask him what he said. Mark became silent once again. The therapist tried engaging Mark and encouraging him but to no avail. The therapist then returned to his paperwork. Mark started crying again and whining something. Again, the therapist attempted to respond to this, with the same result. This was repeated for approximately one hour until, in a barely audible, whiny whisper, Mark said, "Mommy." The therapist praised Mark's accomplishment, told him next time it would be easier to talk, and rewarded Mark by immediately taking him to his mother, who had been instructed ahead of time to praise his actions. Mark was further told that he would be seen in two days and, at that time, he would need to say more than one word in the session.

Mark was slow to become more verbal in subsequent sessions. Initially, each new word was difficult for Mark, was barely audible, and was produced only in response to therapeutic interventions. Mark brought in pictures and toys but at first would not tell the therapist about them or what he wanted to do. The therapist finally told him that if he couldn't say yes or no about doing something, they wouldn't be able to play. The therapist took out a toy Mark had brought and asked if he wanted to play with it. Mark shook his head no. The therapist told Mark he could not understand him unless Mark could verbally tell the therapist. Mark very quietly said "no". The therapist quickly decided to use humor to further the therapeutic alliance. He acted as if he were horrified and said in a humorous way, "You stubbed your toe? Where?!" The therapist then proceeded to grab one of Mark's feet. Mark laughed and said "no" much louder. The therapist would continue to find using humor a useful technique in treating Mark. Humor allowed Mark to interact in a playful, childlike manner and, thus, abandon his guarded, controlling silence. Humor further allowed Mark to enjoy being with the therapist while firm expectations were being set.

As Mark became more comfortable with talking during sessions, oral reading was introduced using a book he was studying in school, and which he had already been able to read aloud to his mother. Again, this started out slowly and almost inaudibly. His efforts and abilities were praised and he appeared proud of himself. It was useful to introduce reading early on in the therapy, as it was planned to use reading as a logical extension to verbal behavior at school.

As the therapist continued treating Mark, his mother reported that he told her he had bad guys in his head and they were keeping him from talking. When the therapist initiated a discussion of the mother's report with Mark, he confirmed this fantasy. As therapy continued, Mark began to tell the therapist that the bad guys in his head were disappearing and being replaced by good guys who allowed him to be comfortable with talking.

Mark enjoyed coming to the sessions and Mrs. Wilson reported improvement in the home and community with a decrease in Mark's temper tantrums and an improved capacity to enjoy himself. She further reported that Mark said, "I like my doctor. He is an adult who can act like a child." This appeared to confirm that Mark was comfortable in the sessions and enjoyed interacting in a less controlled, more childlike manner.

In Mark's case, he required the therapist's direct participation in the school setting. The therapist planned to speak with Mark initially alone and then to have Mark speak with the teacher and classmates. Initially, Mark refused to accompany the therapist out of the classroom. He was then informed of his choices in the situation, which were that he either accompany the therapist on his own initiative, or the therapist would intervene to the extent of physically carrying him out of the classroom, if necessary.

Mark would not come with the therapist, so the therapist followed through and picked Mark up and carried him out of the room. Once out of the room Mark said, "Put me down, I'll walk." He then showed the therapist to a private room where he talked and played for a short period of time. He read his particular practice story for the therapist and then the therapist told him that it was time to read it for the teacher, but to pretend that she was not there at first. The teacher then entered the room but Mark would not read the story. After a short period of time, the teacher left and Mark told the therapist that he was mad at himself but was never reading again. The therapist told Mark that he would have another chance next week when the therapist would return to the school to help him once again. Mark, after much initial refusal, agreed that he would try again next week.

Prior to the therapist's return to the school, the therapist worked with Mark to practice the story, explore his fears, support his previous verbal accomplishments, and discuss the fact that this time when the therapist went to the school, Mark and he would not leave the school until Mark had read for his teacher. Mark was angry about this plan and told the therapist so repeatedly. At times he told the therapist he would never talk to him again and he would never read again. However, using a combination of humor, support, encouragement, and firm limit setting, the therapist was successful in getting Mark to agree to attempt to read in front of his teacher once again. The therapist returned to the school the next week. After receiving help reading the first word of the preselected story, Mark began reading quietly for the teacher. As Mark read, the therapist slowly repositioned the book so Mark was reading directly to the teacher. Once Mark completed his reading, the teacher asked him some preselected questions about colors, and Mark was able to answer her directly. Mark was reinforced verbally by the therapist and received his previously promised special toy surprise. This was a small stuffed animal with a watch attached (a watchdog). This had been carefully selected based on Mark's use of stuffed animals in therapy to express his feelings. Further, his teacher greatly praised his accomplishment. The therapist then left the school and the teacher brought Mark back to his class.

Mark read out loud to one additional child each day until he had read for the entire class. Mark then was required to increase his verbal behaviors by slowly beginning to answer attendance call and then answering preselected questions in front of the class.

When the therapist attempted to begin family therapy, the therapist was told by the family that Mr. Wilson often would not be able to attend sessions because of work. Further, he would not actively take part in the treatment or treatment suggestions. Efforts were made to engage Mr. Wilson in the therapeutic work by scheduling an evening appointment with Mr. Wilson and Mark approximately once per month. Through these appointments, Mr. Wilson became more involved and expressed feelings that in the past he had felt "left out" of the family.

In family sessions it was discovered that each family member would talk for Mark if he was in an uncomfortable situation. Mark might whisper his needs into a family member's ear in a public place and the family member would then respond, allowing Mark to avoid verbal interactions with nonfamily members. The Wilsons recognized this maladaptive response and began to set appropriate limits in this regard. They informed Mark that if he wanted something he needed to ask. This seems to be a simple, logical intervention; however, it was very difficult for the Wilsons to carry out and they were able to do so only after the family's dynamics and their facilitation of Mark's silence were worked through in family therapy sessions.

Therapist: Mark is now speaking fairly easily in sessions and in school, and I wanted to make sure Mark received much of the credit for this because, as you know, it was not always this easy for him. But Mark couldn't have done it without you, because your support and attention mean everything to him, as you are the most important people in his life.

Mother: We are very proud of Mark speaking, but he still has a hard time talking when we go out.

Father: Just the other day we went to the mall and then stopped to get some lunch and Mark wouldn't talk.

Therapist: Really? Mark, what happened?

Mark: I just didn't want to talk.

Therapist: What made it so hard to do?

Mark: I don't know.

Therapist: Mr. and Mrs. Wilson, what did you do when Mark didn't talk?

Mother: Nothing. We just ignored him.

Therapist: Okay, but what happened then? Can you go over what occurred in a step-by-step manner?

Mother: Well, we finished shopping and we were all getting hungry so we decided to go get some lunch. Mark wanted to go to Burger King so we went there but he wouldn't talk.

Therapist: So, who ordered the food?

Mother: Well, when we got to the head of the line, Mark whispered in his brother's ear and his brother ordered.

Therapist: Oh. Huh. How did that happen?

Mother: Well, I guess we've all just gotten used to Mark not talking and communicating his needs to other by whispering in our ears.

Therapist: I see. The whole family sort of talks for Mark when he doesn't want to.

Mother: Yes, I guess we do. But if Mark doesn't whisper to us, how will he get what he wants?

Therapist: By talking himself.

Mother: But if he doesn't, what will happen?

Therapist: Well, I guess in this case, Mark wouldn't get his lunch at Burger King, but I bet when both of you let Mark know by your words and actions that he needs to communicate for himself, otherwise he won't get the things he wants, he will start talking. Is everybody ready to help Mark get over this next hurdle?

Mother: You're sure this won't hurt Mark?

Therapist: Absolutely not. He'll do great. He might miss a meal here or there or not get an ice cream cone or a treat that he wants, but as soon as he gets the idea that you're serious, things will work themselves out. It is important, though, once you set a limit, you must stick with it, even if Mark tries to wear you down like he has in the past.

Father: I'm ready to try it.

Therapist: How about you, Mrs. Wilson?

Mother: I'll do anything to help Mark.

Therapist: Good. Let's set up a plan to help get this started. Mark, I know you love ice cream, so I am going to ask your parents to take you and your brother out for ice cream later on this week, but you'll need to order for yourself if you want ice cream. Okay?

Mark: No, I won't.

Therapist: Okay. Then I guess you really didn't want that ice cream as much as I thought. Mr. and Mrs. Wilson, why don't you try that and we'll talk about what happened at the next appointment. Any questions?

> Mother: No, I think I know what we have to do and I think we can do it.
>
> Therapist: Good. Remember, what you're doing is going to really help Mark to get his mutism under control. Mark, I know this might be hard for you, but remember at first talking with me was very hard and then talking at school was very hard but you were able to do both of those things and look what's happened since then: you made a lot of new friends at school, you're having a lot more fun, and Mom and Dad are very proud of you. It might be hard at first, but I know you can do it. Mr. and Mrs. Wilson, Mark, I will plan on seeing you next week after you've gotten yourself that ice cream cone.

The Wilsons were further instructed to reward verbal behavior and ignore nonverbal behavior. At first, Mark protested, and did not ask for ice cream and thus did not receive any. He further attempted to test the Wilsons' resolve wherever he could but gradually he began being verbal in public places.

Additionally, six months into treatment, Mark's mother revealed that she would occasionally use silence when angry. Mark was described as paying attention but not appearing overly upset by it. This issue was then explored and worked through in the therapy.

Mark continued to talk about the bad guys and good guys in his head. The therapist introduced puppet play with Mark, creating a puppet character who refused to talk. The therapist asked Mark why the puppet wasn't talking and what could be done to help him. Mark slowly began talking about the puppet's fear of talking and having other people laugh at him and hate him. These fears were explored with Mark and he was given support and interpretations within the metaphor of the puppets.

During termination Mark's mother related, "He is a different child. The whole family has noticed. He seems happier and more confident and he hasn't had a temper tantrum in six months. He is still stubborn and hesitant around new people and new situations, but that is Mark."

COMMENTS

Mark's case illustrates a particularly treatment-resistant child and family, but as such it illustrates some important points. Mark's ambivalence about his symptom became clear during the treatment as he was able, with the therapist and his family's help, to extricate himself from the cage his symptom had become. The mutism itself, as well as the control Mark was able to exercise over his family and teachers because of it, were seriously impairing Mark's development. It should also be noted that even in a child whose elective mutism was as family entrenched as Mark's, there was no symptom substitution or detrimental effect from treatment.

SUMMARY

A treatment approach for elective mutism developed at Hawthorn Center (Wright 1968) has been described and illustrated in this chapter. Underlying this approach is the realization that, despite the child's resistance, the child is very ambivalent about his symptoms. The child at some level realizes through this treatment approach that the therapist, unlike previous people in his life including parents, friends, teachers, and relatives, will not give in to his symptom. This is at some level comforting to the child, because it acknowledges the child's ambivalent feelings about not speaking while at the same time supporting his drive toward developmental progress and mastery. The child falls into being silent for many reasons. However, he has found that while it often provides tremendous secondary gains and a sense of power and control, he is frightened by having such power and control over significant adults. The child yearns to shout and scream, to play like other children, and to take part in social activities, but he finds he cannot extricate himself from his current situation. The firm approach the therapist takes in treatment is understood and at some level welcomed by the child. A positive relationship between therapist and child develops as treatment progresses. It is perhaps because of this that at Hawthorn Center, some elective mutes have returned to talk with their therapists years later when facing an unrelated difficult or traumatic situation. This illustrates the strength of the therapeutic alliance formed during the treatment of these children.

It is this therapeutic alliance that is the foundation of the Hawthorn Center approach. It allows these children to side with the healthy part of themselves that wants to play and speak as a normal child. When this has occurred, the feelings of needing to remain in control of themselves and their world through their mutism are no longer necessary.

REFERENCES

American Psychiatric Association (1994). *Diagnostic and Statistical Manual of Mental Disorders, Fourth Edition (DSM-IV)*. Washington, DC: American Psychiatric Association.

Black, B., and Uhde, T. W. (1992). Elective mutism as a variant of social phobia. *Journal of the American Academy of Child and Adolescent Psychiatry* 6:1090–1094.

Brown, J. B., and Lloyd, H. (1975). A controlled study of children not speaking at school. *Journal of Associated Workers of Maladjusted Children* 3:49–63.

Browne, E., Wilson, V., and Laybourne, P. C. (1963). Diagnosis and treatment of elective mutism in children. *Journal of the American Academy of Child Psychiatry* 2:605–617.

Fundudis, T., Kolvin, I., and Garside, R. (1979). *Speech Retarded and Deaf Children: Their Psychological Development*. London: Academic Press.

Hayden, T. L. (1980). Classification of elective mutism. *Journal of the American Academy of Child and Adolescent Psychiatry* 19:118–133.

Kolvin, I., and Fundudis, T. (1981). Elective mute children: psychological development and background factors. *Journal of Child Psychology and Psychiatry* 22:219–232.

Krohn, D., Weckstein, S., and Wright, H. (1992). A study of the effectiveness of a specific treatment for elective mutism. *Journal of the American Academy of Child and Adolescent Psychiatry* 31:711–718.

Kussmaul, A. (1877). *Die Storungen der Sprache*. Leipzig: F. C. W. Vogel.

Labbe, E. E., and Williamson, D. A. (1984). Behavioral treatment of elective mutism: a review of the literature. *Clinical Psychology Review* 4:273–294.

Parker, E. B., Elsen, T. F., and Throckmorton, M. C. (1960). Social casework with elementary school children who do not talk in school. *Social Work* 5:64–70.

Rutter, M. (1977). Delayed speech. In *Child Psychiatry: Modern Approaches*, ed. M. Rutter and L. Hersov, pp. 698–716. Oxford: Blackwell Scientific.

Sanok, R. L., and Ascione, F. R. (1979). Behavioral interventions for elective mutism: an evaluative review. *Child Behavior Therapy* 1:49–67.

Sanok, R. L., and Striefels, S. (1979). Elective mutism: generalization of verbal responding across people and settings. *Behavior Therapy* 10:357–371.

Tramer, M. (1934). Elektiver mutismus be: kindern. *Zeitschriftfur Kinder Psychiatrie* 1:30–35.

Wergeland, H. (1979). Elective mutism. *Acta Psychiatrica Scandinavica* 59:218–228.

Wilkins, R. (1985). A comparison of elective mutism and emotional disorders in children. *British Journal of Psychiatry* 146:198–203.

Wright, H. H., Miller, M. D., Cook, M. A., and Lihman, J. R. (1985). Early identification and intervention with children who refuse to speak. *Journal of the American Academy of Child Psychiatry* 24:739–746.

Wright, H. L. (1968). A clinical study of children who refuse to talk in school. *Journal of the American Academy of Child Psychiatry* 7:603–617.

16

"SPEECH IS SILVERN, BUT SILENCE IS GOLDEN":[1] DAY HOSPITAL TREATMENT OF TWO ELECTIVELY MUTE CHILDREN

Eleanor Barrett Krolian

REVIEW OF THE LITERATURE

The diagnostic entity known as elective mutism describes a symptom picture that is rarely seen, faintly if ever heard, and until recently infrequently written about in the American child psychiatry literature.

The first reference to this disorder was by the German physician Kussmaul in 1877. He used the term *aphasia voluntaria* to describe mentally sound people who refused to speak. Over the course of time it was variously known as "speech inhibition" (Chapin and Corcoran 1947), "psychogenic mutism" (Mitscherlich 1961), or "thymogetic mutism" (Waterink and Vedder 1936). In 1934, Tramer coined the term *elective mutism* to describe those children who, in selected settings and with selected people, choose not to speak. This is the diagnostic appellation that is now generally used.

---

1. See Meyer Zeligs (1961) for a brief history of this saying, the first half of which has been dropped from common usage.

The electively mute child is one who, while possessing the proven ability to speak and understand language, exhibits partial speech avoidance. In the majority of cases the child speaks freely to family members and within the confines of the home. Once outside the home, however, these children become steadfastly silent and maintain their muteness in the face of enticements, threats, criticism, and peer pressure. The muteness pervades almost all social interactions outside the boundary of home and family.

Electively mute children are described as characteristically immature (Halpern et al. 1971) and as controlling and oppositional. In observing their behavior one often feels in the presence of an obstinate 2-year-old who may not say "no" but exudes negativism in most of his or her actions. The electively mute child is also characterized as "slow to warm up" to use Thomas and colleagues' (1968) term. Frequently, they manifest problems of bladder or bowel control. Kolvin and Fundudis (1981) report that in their sample of 24 elective mutes, 42 percent were enuretic and 17 percent were encopretic.

When one first encounters these children, their vacant and withdrawn look is striking. Eye contact is avoided and it is an arduous task to assess the child's affective state since so little is offered by way of facial expression or body gestures and of course there are no words to help anchor our diagnostic thoughts.

The symptom generally first presents itself when the child enters a school setting (Elson et al. 1965). The range in age of onset is usually from 3 to 5 years (Salfield 1950), though some authors report onset as late as 7 years (Goll 1979). It is only slightly more common in girls and the prevalence in the general population is quite low, with some authors reporting the incidence to be as low as 0.5 percent (Bradley and Sloman 1975, Reed 1963). Prior to the child's school entrance many parents at first report no abnormalities in the use of spontaneous speech or the quality of social relatedness in the child. On closer investigation, however, one often uncovers longstanding pockets of excessive shyness pointing to the possibility of an insidious rather than acute onset of the symptom.

It is no coincidence that the appearance of the symptom frequently coincides with the child's first major move out of the family system. Several authors refer to separation and abandonment issues (Browne et al. 1963), the intense mutual dependency between mother and child (Halpern et al. 1971, von Misch 1952), and the isolated and closed nature of the mutist's family (Goll 1979, Halpern et al. 1971) in examining the etiological factors of the disorder. That separation difficulties frequently accompany a diagnosis of elective mutism was borne out in one of the patients described in this chapter.

In establishing the differential diagnosis for elective mutism Browne and her co-authors (1963) state that other disorders or conditions in which mutism is found should be ruled out. These include mental retardation, schizophrenia, aphasia, hearing loss, and hysterical aphonia. In one case report by Kummer (1953), a child's mutism was related to hypothyroidism and a treatment with hormonal replacement therapy was successful in alleviating the mutism. The literature reveals a difference of opinion on the role of organic factors and articulation difficulties in these children. Kehrer and Tinkl-Damhorst (1974), for example, include organically determined speech defects and brain damage under the rubric "elective mutism." As yet there are no definitive studies that rule out these factors in formulating the diagnosis. There is also divergence on whether or not elective mutism is a neurotic reaction or a disturbance of personality as reported by some authors (Browne et al. 1963, Chethik 1973, Pustrom and Speers 1964, Spieler 1944).

Part of the difficulty in producing accurate statistical research on these children is the floating parameters used among authors to describe the disorder. There are divergent opinions on the duration and scope of the mutism, etiology, inclusion of non–English-speaking children in samples, age of onset, and neurological factors. Though elective mutism appears as a separate diagnostic entity in *DSM-III*, there is still debate as to whether it is a symptom connected with other specific disorders such as "oppositional disorder," whether it is a clear and distinct diagnostic classification, or whether it is a symptom that cuts across various diagnostic categories. Other factors confounding the research are the very low prevalence of the disorder in the general society and the fact that many studies do not use adequate control groups for comparison.

However, when the families of elective mutes are examined there are consistent findings noted in several areas. There is a higher incidence of family pathology and/or marital disharmony than in control groups. Kolvin and Fundudis (1981) report that 58 percent of the families of twenty-four electively mute children they studied showed some combination of parental pathology, family pathology, or marital discord. A number of cases reviewed reported maternal depression (Chethik 1973, Kolvin and Fundudis 1981).

Almost all authors reviewed point to a symbiotic relationship between mother and child in which the child is often controlling and abusive of the parent. The push for the symbiotic tie is fueled by the mother's dissatisfaction with the marital relationship or the actual absence of the father from the home. (The latter is the case in both of the patients to be described.) The mothers of elective mutes are often described as "immature" (Mora and colleagues 1962) and many never leave the home of their family of origin (Wright 1968). Some of these mothers have never worked outside the home. In addition, these families show varying degrees of social dysfunction. Many are economically unstable (Adams and Glasner 1954), socially isolated (Parker et al. 1960), and are suspicious of those outside the immediate family (Goll 1979).

In one of the only detailed theories on how the family of the elective mute child functions, the Swedish author Goll (1979) offers an elaborate description of the role playing that occurs within the families of these children. His premise is that these families have very little confidence in society and therefore insulate themselves from all forms of contact outside the family. The crisis occurs when the child must step out of this closed system into the society that the family has taught him to distrust. His loyalty to the family outweighs the pressure to interact with strangers and the mutism unfolds.

There have been several other conceptual frameworks offered regarding the etiology of the symptom. Some authors espouse the theory of a family neurosis (Browne et al. 1963). Others believe that the child experienced a traumatic event at the time of speech development (Parker et al. 1960), perhaps an assault of some sort to the mouth. Still other authors note that the symptom is a synthesis of conflicts from all phases of psychosexual development (Chethik 1973). As a neurotic symptom, the mutism could be seen as an oral conflict characterized by overdependency, an anal conflict expressed by the stubborn withholding of speech, or a phallic conflict over sexual excitement and mastery (Weissman 1982).

I would suggest that a closer look must also be given to the quality of the mother–child interaction during the period of language acquisition and speech formation in the first two years of life. Bruner (1966) notes that the "ritualized reciprocal mother–child interchanges in play provide the context for drawing the child's attention to communication, to the form that communication takes and to the mother's words themselves." Miller (1979) suggests that the "acquisition of language, through its external manifestation as speech, derives from the need for closeness in the face of the ongoing separation-individuation process by being an internalization of the caretaking person and by being an avenue of communicative contact" (p. 135).

Thus, when a child's speech is disrupted at the time of an actual separation from the parent, it may indicate a past failure to develop a reciprocal communication pattern between mother and child at the very first phases of the separation–individuation process. Instead of object loss and internalization spurring on the development of language, we see the child revert to a regressed level of preverbal communication in order to maintain oneness with and infantile dependence upon the object.

Further, if there is maternal depression, as has been reported in a significant number of electively mute families, then language development is further hindered. As Edgcumbe (1981) points out, "achieving gratification of wishes via interaction with the object is an important motive for language development which is lost or diminished if the object is unresponsive" (p. 100). An early maternal depression can set the stage then for subsequent pathology in the area of speech development and use.

A further point that requires more study is the actual level of language development in the mothers of these children. In both cases that I will report the mothers show an impoverished use of language. Their speech is sparse and unspontaneous. There is no richness of affect, form, or content. They generally show no change in intonation or modulation of speech regardless of the content being expressed, and one gains little sense of their feeling state. Both parents are from low socioeconomic backgrounds.

A variety of treatment approaches for these children is found in the literature. Behaviorists suggest treating elective mutism as a phobia and using stimulus-fading techniques or increasingly coercive means to extinguish the behavior (Halpern et al. 1971). Family therapists find justification for collaborative family therapy along with individual treatment of the child to gain beneficial therapeutic results (Goll 1979). Psychoanalysis is shown to be effective (Chethik 1973), and persuasive arguments are also made for removal of the child from the pathological family by placing him or her in institutional or inpatient hospital care (Amman 1958, Goll 1979). The treatment approaches run the gamut from those that address the symptom alone to those that explore the underlying conflict.

The only consensus about treatment one finds in the literature is that individual therapy with the child alone is the least successful of the therapeutic interventions. This finding supports the notion that the family is involved in the development and maintenance of the symptom. It also supports several authors' contention that the symptom is fairly intractable and requires intensive therapeutic effort (Halpern et al. 1971, Salfield 1950, Yates 1970).

In this review I found only one article that presented day treatment of these children. In this article by Halpern and his co-workers (1971), the authors report only their behavioral approach to alleviating the symptom in the three cases reported. They refer only briefly to the family treatment and there is no indication that any individual psychotherapy with the children was undertaken.

It is interesting to note that several of the authors who report improvement in the symptom picture after treatment also note that the child failed to ever speak a word in the treatment situation (Chethik 1973, Ruzicka and Sackin 1974). Pustrom and Speers (1964) view this sustained silence in the treatment setting as the child's last effort to retain omnipotent control of others. Chethik (1973), in his analysis of a 6½-year-old electively mute girl, is careful to point out that with such patients the level of ego functioning that is achieved is not without conflict, and therefore is subject to regression when under stress, particularly, for example, when entering adolescence.

In the follow-up studies reviewed, differing results were reported and some conclusions appear to be equivocal. Elson and colleagues (1965) report "very encouraging" findings after a six-month to five-year follow-up study of four electively mute children treated on an inpatient setting. Though positive findings were reported, they included the absence of sociopathic behavior, depressive symptoms, and sleep disturbance, none of which had been reported as present before treatment. A significant improvement in speech was reported, but only two of the four children performed better academically, all continued to have impaired peer relations (though better than prehospitalization), one patient showed a possible thought disorder, and no improvement in the family pathology was reported. Interestingly, though the authors were encouraged by their results, the mothers of these children as a whole did not perceive increased verbalization as a sign of success of the treatment.

Wergeland's (1979) follow-up study of eleven children diagnosed as electively mute concluded that five children who received no treatment were better adjusted than those who were separated from their families and hospitalized for treatment. Of the four children treated in the hospital, three relinquished their mutism but two were later diagnosed as neurotic and one as psychotic. Two children who received outpatient treatment remained unchanged during the treatment.

The prognostic picture for these children is one of serious concern. As would be expected, a poorer prognosis exists for those cases in which there are multiple problems, such as thought disorders, low intelligence, and neurologic impairment (Kupietz and Schwartz 1982).

Additionally, Hayden (1980) found that spontaneous remission with age is rare in electively mute children, and the presence of the symptom through adolescence is frequently accompanied by behavior in the prepsychotic to psychotic range. One could speculate that the symptom, when carried into adolescence, is associated with more serious pathology, such as a weak ego structure that is not capable of withstanding the developmental tasks of adolescence, especially the task of separating from family.

It is obvious from these reviews that no consensus has been reached on the course and prognosis of elective mutism. More long-term follow-up on these children is clearly needed. There is also debate about whether the presence or eventual removal of the symptom itself is useful in determining prognosis, or whether the underlying pathology is the real determinant of long-term adjustment for these children.

These children are among the most challenging and thought-provoking to treat. They test our very therapeutic mettle by not dealing in the tender of our trade—words. They sit silently in front of you, eyes averted, unmoving, and they wait. You may suggest something they'd like to play with, but odds are there will be no reply. You may even venture a comment on their sad look, but it will seem to fall on deaf ears. The therapist is left hearing his or her own voice and does not know at first if he or she has been heard, confirmed, or denied. Clearly, the soil is rich for countertransference reactions to these children.

Therapists must be mindful, then, of several significant issues in taking on the treatment of an electively mute child. First and foremost, we must be keenly aware of our reaction to the prolonged silence of the child. We must be aware of the feeling of impotence and anger and the wish, so to speak, to be the one who "gets the goose to lay the golden egg." Furthermore, if the silence is experienced primarily as a resistance, the treatment will not move.

Second, as Kahn (1963) so beautifully points out in his analysis of a silent 18-year-old boy, silence is a communication. It must be listened to, experienced, and understood as an expression of the patient's past experience and conflicts. Arlow (1961) and Zeligs (1961) note that silence in analysis serves the purpose of discharge, defense, and communication, and I believe the same applies to the silence of the elective mute. Blos (1972) offers an interpretation of the silence of an analytic patient that poignantly captures the quality of the silence that I have experienced in working with these children. He wrote, "Words are intrusive and also emphasize separateness. The silence is an acting out of an earlier time when life was good and union with the object was felt as possible. It is also an identification with a mother who had been silent at a critical time." A third concern in the treatment of these children is how the therapist actually negotiates the withholding silence. Glover (1955) warns against the "pugilistic encounter" in which the therapist counters the patient's silence with his or her own. Conversely, therapists may be so distressed by the deafening and frustrating silence of these children that, without adequate therapeutic thought or reason, they fill in the silence themselves, thus compromising their empathetic attunement to the child. Related to this, Chethik (1973) addresses the technical problems in making interpretations to these children. He warns against making interpretations that are based on the therapist's constructions and not adequately substantiated by material from the patient. He also notes that correct interpretations can create problems in that the child feels his or her mind and innermost thoughts are being read by the omniscient therapist and this can lead to undue anxiety.

One must also avoid reproach, which can lead to devaluation of the silence and an overvaluation of speech. For these children speech truly is silvern and silence is golden.

Though there remain many open questions about etiology, prognosis, and optimal treatment strategies for these children, and indeed whether elective mutism should be considered as a separate diagnosis at all rather than as a symptom, some well-considered hypotheses can be offered to the reader at this point.

Both this writer's experience and much of the literature support the position that children with varying levels of ego development and varying degrees of learning problems carry a primary diagnosis of elective mutism. The degree of psychopathology seems to span from the severely neurotically disturbed child to the child with extreme borderline features in his or her personality development. These children often show neuropsychological difficulties such as learning disabilities that the mutism may initially mask. In the cases to be presented here, one child exhibited a separation anxiety with many oppositional and negativistic features, while the second child was seen as a poorly integrated borderline youngster with profoundly impaired object relations. Both children had low intelligence (borderline to low average) with mild to moderate learning disabilities.

The dynamic reason for the choice of this symptom over others can be traced back preliminarily to the mother–child relationship, specifically the aspect of attuned reciprocal communication in the dyad. In both of the cases to be discussed, the mothers of these children presented with a marked verbal constriction, rare spontaneous speech, and a general absence of affect and eye contact when interacting with others. The symptom in the child functions as a means of maintaining a primary identification with and dependence upon this unresponsive, unattuned, and, I would venture, very frequently depressed mother. It allows the child to preserve a tenacious but ambivalent tie to the object with the hope of eventual union. When the child is old enough to leave home for the first time, the expressed "loyalty" to mother can be maintained by excluding other significant adults through silence, which may also permit the displaced expression of aggression against the ungiving mother. The regressive quality of the return to a preverbal level should not be underestimated when assessing the actual level of ego functioning in these children. It is clearly a symptom that seriously affects the child's ability to develop socially, academically, and psychologically.

DESCRIPTION OF THE CHILDREN'S DAY HOSPITAL

Before presenting the two cases, a brief description of the Children's Day Hospital will provide the reader with an understanding of the special milieu in which the treatment of these children took place.

The Children's Day Hospital at New York Hospital, Westchester Division, provides a broad range of services for grammar school–age children whose emotional and educational needs warrant an intensive setting in which special education and comprehensive psychiatric care are provided within the framework of an integrated treatment milieu. Services are available for the duration of the grade-school years so that long-term treatment is possible, if indicated. The program continues through the summer, as well as during all school vacations, so that the intensive treatment services can operate year round, without interruption.

Each child in the program receives a full evaluation, leading to the development of an individualized treatment plan. Therapeutic modalities include individual, group, and family therapy; psychotropic medication, as indicated; behavior modification within the context of the therapeutic milieu; art therapy; recreational therapy; and occupational therapy, with an emphasis on prevocational preparation. Education takes place in small class settings (maximum of five children per class), with individualization of the educational approaches and goals for each child, and ample one-to-one support available.

An interdisciplinary team approach is utilized so that treatment can be well coordinated and integrated into the child's daily routine. The staff includes child psychiatrists; a consulting pediatric neurologist; psychologists; social workers; special education teachers; a speech and language consultant; psychiatric nurses; art, recreation, and occupational therapists; and mental health counselors.

Children eligible for the day hospital have emotional disturbances that interfere with participation in an ordinary classroom setting. These include children with a wide variety of psychiatric disorders such as childhood depression, hyperactivity, conduct disorders, borderline personality organization, avoidance reactions, psychotic disorders, and elective mutism. Frequently, these emotional disturbances are complicated by learning disabilities, neurological dysfunction, and dysfunction in the family. These complications are addressed within the overall treatment program.

It is my opinion that day hospital care offers a unique opportunity for the long-term intensive therapeutic intervention that is required to produce lasting change in these children. Day treatment stands as a viable alternative to removing these children from their homes, a move that I do not feel is always as clinically indicated as some authors would have us believe.

A day hospital setting can become an arena that gradually and nonintrusively encourages interaction between the child and staff and the child and peers by its consistent, supportive, and stable nature. Slowly, the predictable nature of the staff and milieu, in conjunction with the specific therapies applied, helps move the child from an unrelated and withdrawn position to a point where an interest is sparked in finding out about these new people that populate his or her world. It also allows an optimal distance to work on the symbiotic tie between mother and child.

CASE HISTORY: PAUL

Paul was an 8-year, 1-month-old boy at the time of his admission to the day hospital. He had received five months of outpatient psychotherapy, initiated by his school district, for his refusal to speak in school and severe separation anxiety, which prevented him from attending school without his mother. When these symptoms did not remit to outpatient treatment, a referral for more intensive day hospital treatment followed.

Paul was the younger of two boys born into this African-American, lower-class family. His mother, Ms. A., was 18 years old at the time of birth and had not maintained a relationship with Paul's father, and Paul has never had contact with him.

Ms. A.'s pregnancy with Paul progressed without prenatal care as she concealed her condition from her family until shortly before giving birth. Upon delivery, she intended to surrender her son for adoption but was vehemently opposed in this by the maternal grandmother. Ms. A. passively acceded and brought her unwanted son home.

Developmental milestones were essentially within normal limits. Ms. A. could recount little about her son's temperament or what type of infant and toddler he was to parent. It appeared as if, affectively, she took little notice of him until at age 2 he began to display what she termed temper tantrums. The behavior she described her son exhibiting seemed within normal bounds for the developmental phase but was apparently significantly taxing enough for her to take notice.

Symptomatic behavior was noticed just before Paul's fourth birthday. He began to attend a preschool program and would not speak a word to anyone there. He clung excessively to his mother and cried out her name at night. This behavior increased when Ms. A. was hospitalized for a tubal ligation on Paul's fourth birthday. He feared that she would not return from the hospital. When she did return he would not let her out of his sight and insisted on sleeping with her at night. He also began to experience some confusion between his maternal aunt and mother, referring to his aunt as "Mommy" and calling his mother by her given name.

The A. family was a tightly knit, socially isolated household dominated by the maternal grandmother. The family kept to themselves and there was a great deal of interdependence among the members (both familial factors that may have added to Paul's choice of isolating silence as a symptom). The household was composed of both maternal grandparents, Ms. A. and her two sons, and one of Ms. A.'s two sisters. The other sister lived nearby and was in close contact with the family. Ms. A.'s self-description was of a Cinderella-like role in her family and she never felt that she withstood the comparisons to her two college-educated and employed sisters. Paul's mother had attended but never graduated from high school, briefly held two menial jobs, and had never lived apart from her family of origin.

Ms. A. was an extremely overweight and burdened young woman who was affectively totally unexpressive and responded in the most limited verbal way to questions. She had a long history of clinical depression and at various points had sought outpatient psychiatric treatment. When Paul was 3 years old, she made a suicide attempt with an overdose of Valium. When Paul was 10 she again contemplated suicide after the death of a very close relative. Ms. A. had described this relative as "the only person I could talk to." She refused all therapeutic interventions offered to her at that time.

Of her relationship with Paul, Ms. A. stated that she eventually "grew to like him," though obviously never making a close connection to him. Within the family, Paul was overindulged and regularly given his own way, which fostered areas of obstinate, controlling, and regressive behavior. As late as Paul's seventh year his grandmother reported that he would refuse to wipe himself after a bowel movement and would scream until his mother came to assist him. Though Ms. A. occasionally expressed the wish to live on her own with her sons and separate from her family, she also feared that she might hurt her sons if left alone to parent them.

Collaborative work with this family was very difficult to maintain, and in fact, there was an inverse relationship between their involvement and Paul's mutism. For example, Ms. A. and her parents refused to keep a single appointment once Paul began to talk freely in the day hospital. Their reasoning was that if Paul was doing so well, the family did not need to meet with the staff. It appeared that the family unconsciously experienced Paul's verbal communicativeness as an abandonment and rejection of the isolated and circumscribed family system.

After admission to the day hospital, a neurological examination was performed that was essentially within normal limits except for difficulties in higher integrative functions, suggestive of mild learning disabilities. Psychological testing was attempted, but Paul's complete refusal to cooperate prevented any assessment of intelligence, personality, and neuropsychological functioning.

Though Paul remained essentially silent on the unit for twelve months, there was always an engaging quality about him that permitted peers and staff to weather his long silence. The absence of his verbal communication never left one feeling that Paul was unrelated to what went on around him, and he often evoked in others the desire to reach out to him. The impression was of a child with near-normal capacity for object relations if the mutism could be lifted.

CASE HISTORY: ANN

Ann was 7½ years old on admission to the day hospital. She had a history of electively mute behavior in preschool and school settings dating to her third year when she first entered a preschool program. She was mute in kindergarten, but spoke limitedly in a therapeutic nursery program in the same year. First grade was spent in a small special education classroom where, again, she was silent. Her teacher observed that Ann often wanted to speak but would hold herself back, sometimes by biting her hand or putting an object into her mouth. While in the first grade, Ann began outpatient psychotherapy and continued for several months. During the course of the treatment, she spoke only twice to the therapist, once stating, "The devil's inside me and I'm going to get you." Her therapist was impressed by Ann's determined hold on her silence and her blunted affect. He felt that the possibility of a thought disorder could not be ruled out and that beneath the mutism was a great deal of unexpressed aggression.

Past history revealed that Ms. T., Ann's mother, was 20 years old at the time of Ann's birth. She developed toxemia at term and labor was induced. Ann's birth weight was 4 lb., 1 oz. and her Apgar score was 5–7. She required two weeks' incubation before being released from the hospital in good condition.

Motor development revealed that Ann sat at 6½ months, walked alone at 11 months, and said single words at less than a year. Though reported to be an average eater and to have had no feeding problems, Ann was a smaller than average baby, weighing only 10 lbs. at 6½ months.

Ann was the oldest of three daughters born to her single, black mother. The middle sister was born when Ann was 2 (a year before she began preschool), and Ann displayed only mild jealousy toward this sibling. The youngest sister was born when Ann was 8. Prior to the onset of the mutism, Ms. T. reported no indications of excessive shyness, withholding of speech, or withdrawn behavior. Ann evidenced no difficulty in separating from her mother.

Ms. T. was an obese, withdrawn, and depressed-looking young

woman who maintained only fleeting eye contact and spoke most sparingly. She described herself as being quite shy as a youngster, though never mute. Her answers to the most detailed questions were strikingly brief, unrevealing, and delivered without affect. This was especially true when asked to recall qualitative details rather than concrete facts about Ann's growth and development. Though Ms. T. clearly provided ably for Ann's physical needs, her ability to be emotionally attuned to her daughter was limited.

The T. family, like the A. family, functioned as an insulated unit closed off from much contact with the outside world. The family had no phone, so that communicating with them was difficult. Ms. T. had no contact with Ann's father, and Ann reportedly never asked about him. Ann's maternal grandmother lived in a neighboring state but Ms. T. had no contact at all with her, alluding only to the fact that there had been a falling-out in years past. This relationship was so severed that Ann had no knowledge her grandmother even existed. This pattern of severing significant relationships through silence may be a common factor in examining a family predisposition for the symptom choice of elective mutism.

Ann's silence on the unit was quite isolating. She often remained on the periphery of activity and appeared unconnected and uninvolved. Her muteness had a cold and distancing quality to it that often pushed others away, rather than stimulating interest in breaking through the barrier of silence to reach her. She presented as a youngster with severe impairment in object relations whose muteness kept her at increasingly greater distance from establishing normal object ties.

COURSE OF TREATMENT: PAUL

Paul's mutism was complete when he first came to the day hospital, though he was reported to be fully verbal outside school settings. Not only did he not talk in school, but he perfected the silent sneeze, the clandestine cough, and the noiseless belch. For months not a sound could be heard from him. He refused to indicate even his most basic needs such as to go to the bathroom and would end up wetting himself rather than let his need be known. He also showed an extreme separation anxiety disorder that required his mother remain at school with him for several weeks after his admission.

Our initial treatment approach was to allow him some time and room to develop trust of and familiarity with his new surroundings. We did expect that he would respond to questions with a nod or shake of his head and generally he complied. He was seen two times weekly in individual, group, and art therapy. In all three therapy situations he remained completely silent. The first breakthrough of speech occurred one year after admission in weekly sessions with his speech teacher, after she had taught him to use American Sign Language. He first began to sign to his classmates and the speech teacher, and then he offered single-word answers to the speech teacher's questions as he hid under a desk or behind a screen. He began to communicate verbally to his classroom teacher thirteen months after admission after she told him that he could go no further with his reading unless he began to sound out the letters of the alphabet. The two of them began meeting daily in the supply closet and after about five days of showing Paul a flash card with the letter "a" he issued the grunted sound of the letter. Slowly he began to read in the classroom with just the teacher present and right by his side. Gradually she moved her chair away from his desk until she was sitting at her own desk as he read. The teacher then began to ask questions related to the reading material and Paul answered, often with his head covered or eyes averted. By June 1983, Paul would occasionally talk to classmates when the teacher was out of the room and vice versa.

When I undertook Paul's individual treatment in August 1982, I was not sure what to expect. He had not spoken to his previous therapist except to say "Do you want to play hide and seek?" in one of their last sessions together. He had begun to speak sporadically to his case coordinator (the staff member responsible for management of the case), and most of his communications were of an angry and demanding nature. For instance, he once told her that if she wanted to hear him speak, she had better give him hundreds of hours because that was what it would take.

In our first session Paul did not speak a word. He bounded into my office and shut the door so that I could not enter. He then proceeded to hand me all of my belongings—pocketbook, umbrella, and briefcase—as I sat outside the door. I commented that it looked as though I was moving out and he nodded with a satisfied grin. When I asked who was moving in, he pointed to himself with a gleeful smile and slammed the door shut. He was clearly announcing his arrival as well as letting me know who was going to run the show.

From the second session on Paul was fully and fluently verbal. This was six months after he began to utter sounds to his speech teacher. He spoke with the couch pillow covering his face and I must admit that at first I was thankful for his use of the pillow because it allowed me to take notes on his torrent of words and rich fantasy play. As we addressed the purpose of our work together he stated that his goal was "to get out of this funny farm."

There were two factors that contributed to Paul's ability to use free, spontaneous speech at this early point in his treatment. First, Paul had known me for two and a half years as his group therapist, and we therefore had the basis for a therapeutic relationship. Second, Paul was finishing his second year of day hospital treatment and he was also experiencing more internal discomfort and external pressure from peers to speak. I believe that through the heroic preparatory work done with his previous therapists, Paul was now more able to respond both to our therapeutic relationship and to the more ego-dystonic feelings about his mutism, and he began to open up.

There were several themes that surfaced early in our sessions. Paul had a great need to maintain control. He always had to arrive in my office first and then tell me that I could come in. He would demand snacks, extra sessions, or more time. He often wanted to leave the office, for instance to go bowling, which I did not permit, since I felt he was healthy enough to manage his anxiety within the session. He handled this particular frustration of his wish in a most ingenious way. He lay on the couch with his feet up in the air and moved them in an exaggerated walking motion, all the while giving a vivid step-by-step narration of an imaginary trip to the bowling alley and his subsequent embarrassing defeat of me at the lane.

A second theme related to his wish to be invulnerable. He told me of his special bullet-proof vest that protected him even if a Mack truck hit him. With this vest he could jump from a two-story building and not get hurt. The only problem was that his vest ran on Duracell batteries and several times they were precariously close to dying. In this play, he seemed to be attempting to master early feelings of inadequate protection by his often depressed and depleted mother. Phallic strivings could also be seen clearly as he repeatedly told me and assured himself that his car was stronger than mine and that I could never knock his over.

A third theme centered on the role of secrets in the family. In one session Paul presented a whole series of characters who were "ghosts in the closet." There were 1000-year-old grandfather ghosts, 99-year-old father ghosts, and a host of "kid ghosts." As Paul described these ghosts I was warned not to tell anyone in his family about them.

Another early theme related to Paul's difficulty seeing himself as a distinct and separate person with an identity of his own. In his play he created a multitude of interesting and often humorous characters, but they were always called "no name." Slowly these characters gained more substance and became more forceful and finally were given names. One of the more interesting ones was a clever thief named "Hitler Jones," who would abscond with items from my desk but always return them before being caught. Eventually, Paul began to use his own initials to identify his characters.

Two months into treatment, Paul began working directly on his silence. In one session he said that he hated all the people in school. When I asked what he thought would happen if he talked to the staff here, he angrily responded, "They wouldn't say anything." This highlighted both his anal withholding tendencies as well as his fear that significant people in his life would not respond to him. When I later asked what made it possible for him to talk with me, he quickly said, "We'll talk about that in two weeks."

Slowly, Paul began to show concern about the effect his silence had on his functioning. At one point he asked what his grade levels were and I shared with him how far behind he was. He quickly and firmly countered that he could catch up. I agreed with him, but added that talking was what would likely help him catch up the quickest. Paul accepted my intervention though with a certain amount of anxiety. His response was to say "wait a minute" and then after a few seconds, as if he had digested the comment, he told me that I could continue talking. I responded by offering that perhaps in our next session we could think more about how his silence had affected his schoolwork. My decision to move away from this anxiety-producing material follows Pine's (1984) suggestion that with fragile patients, more therapeutic gain can be accomplished when interpretations and interventions are made at a point when the conflict or painful affect is not active. He suggests "striking when the iron is cold" in order "to make the interpretation usable by the patient, who must have adequate control structure to receive it" (pp. 60–61).

Slowly Paul introduced different aspects of his family life into the sessions. He told of special people in his family who liked to do the things he liked. He talked of a favorite teenage cousin who was killed in a car crash but whose birthday he still celebrated. His close and special relationship to his maternal grandfather with whom he went fishing on Sunday afternoons was poignantly described, and he proudly told of how he hoodwinked his grandmother by hiding in the attic when she came to punish him. In his accounts of family life his mother was only fleetingly mentioned and then only on direct question from me. That was the case until one particular session about seven months into treatment. As Paul lounged comfortably on my couch in this session, we talked about sleeping arrangements in the home. He reported that he, his mother, and brother shared a room. I commented that there had been a time when he used to share a bed with his mother and he agreed. I asked if he remembered when it happened that he no longer slept with her. He said that it was when he was 3 or 4 years old and I made the connection that that was about the time he stopped talking. Suddenly Paul was propelled from his luxuriating position on the couch and landed in an astonished heap on the floor. With total surprise he asked, "How did that happen? Somebody kicked me out." I commented to Paul that just as we were talking about his leaving his mother's bed, he got kicked out. He adamantly denied responsibility for his tumble to the floor and added that he didn't get kicked out of his mother's bed. I offered that perhaps "kicked out" was the way a little boy could feel when he had to leave his mother's bed. This interchange opened the door for subsequent discussions of other, actual separations and feelings of distance from his mother. He was able to share sad and then mad feelings that he had at the time of his mother's hospitalization on his fourth birthday. Though he was glad upon her return home, he also admitted not feeling sure that she would stay.

In subsequent sessions, we explored his use of the pillow as a barrier between us when he talked in session. Though it served several different functions including protecting me from his angry feelings, it also represented the barrier to affective communication that existed between Paul as an eager, active infant and his mother as a depressed and unresponsive caregiver. I pointed out to Paul how the pillow prevented him from seeing my facial responses to him and in that way protected him from the same kind of disappointment he felt with his mother.

By January 1983, Paul had managed his first full session without the use of the pillow. His use of speech had begun to overflow the confines of the office. He would say a few words on the way to and from the sessions, and he used the sessions to make actual phone calls to me as I sat in another office. In class and in the milieu there was more generalized use of speech. He started to read aloud in class while his teacher and other students were there, and he also offered answers to direct questions from certain of the nursing staff. In direct correlation to this increase in verbal production was an increase in his oppositional and mildly aggressive behavior. The staff was so pleased to see Paul come to life that we had to be cautious not to permit him behavior that would not be tolerated in other children.

Paul's second summer in the day hospital proved to be a period of the most marked change in his behavior. By the end of July, Paul was talking spontaneously in almost all areas of the program and to both staff and peers. He was becoming a very active and vocal presence in the community and he often required limits on his screaming and cursing. His teacher reported the dilemma that he, the teacher, felt in telling an elective mute to stop talking in class. Paul's self-description was of a "mad bomber" and his forceful spurting out of words and his challenging behavior in class and milieu attested to this description.

In examining what factors in the milieu occurred over the summer that induced his relinquishing the mutism, there are several that deserve mention. First, Paul was increasingly concerned about when he would leave the day hospital. His best friend was leaving the program in the fall and this gave pause for Paul to reflect on his own functioning and I believe it added fire to his progressive developmental push.

Second, during the summer, eight college-age volunteers joined our program and they spent all day with the children. Paul's ego strengths permitted him to take this chance for a fresh beginning with a new group of people who did not know him solely as a mute child. Finally, the admission of Ann in the early summer played a major role in Paul's giving up his mutism. Peers began to tease Paul about his similarity to this frail, silent little girl. He daily rode to and from the program on the bus with her and he had the opportunity to make an objective observation of what his own silence looked like and felt like to others. The symptom became increasingly ego-dystonic and more difficult for him to maintain until finally the floodgates opened and he began to use free, spontaneous, and well-formed speech.

COURSE OF TREATMENT: ANN

Ann was admitted to the unit in June 1983. She, like Paul, was reported to be fully verbal at home, though the reliability of her mother as a reporter was questionable because of her own speech limitations.

On first look Ann appeared shy, withdrawn, and passive. She rather too willingly complied with the procedures of admission and seemed not to care when her mother left her at the program on her first day. In her mental status exam with a female physician, however, Ann's shy passivity was soon replaced with a bold intrusiveness as she silently rifled through the examiner's pockets and desk drawers with an air of defiance and surety.

Within a week after admission, Ann had exhibited some limited use of speech. The situations in which the speech was elicited as well as the content of her communications gave us an understanding of the dynamic factors that contributed to her mutism. First, Ann formed a very quick alliance with an extremely overweight 12-year-old female patient on the unit. In this relationship Ann's use of her silence to obtain infantile gratification could clearly be observed. The 12-year-old patient treated Ann like a mother would treat a very young child. She bounced Ann on her knee, cuddled her in her lap, and preened with joy as Ann began to pass a few whispered words her way. Additionally, certain of the interactions between the two girls had a sadistic flavor and highlighted the secondary gain Ann received from her withholding mutist behavior. For example, the older patient would provocatively tickle or playfully pinch Ann until Ann would say "I love you." Ann clearly enjoyed these interchanges and would invariably come back for more. One can speculate in what way this may be a repetition of what occurs at home.

A second significant occasion of speech occurred the second week after admission. Its significance could be found not only in the content but also in the fact that it was the only time to date that Ann offered clearly distinct and audible speech in conversation form. In this conversation Ann and another female patient engaged in a provocative and graphic sexual discussion of boyfriends. Ann did most of the talking and was quite aggressive in her presentation of this heated material. Staff members overheard this conversation and were struck by both the flood of aggressive and sexual feelings that poured out of Ann and her immediate sealing off and return to silence. We began to see her silence as a not so effective lid on a sea of turbulent drives. This titillating conversation along with her sexualized manner of relating to male staff raised the concern of the possibility of past sexual abuse or exposure to sexual activity, though no history of this has been reported.

Since that time Ann's verbalizations have been rare, whispered comments to one or two female peers. It is of interest to note that she very often produced a clear and loud laugh when she was either enjoying a game or had pulled a prank on someone, especially an adult.

In the classroom Ann was able to perform solidly on a first-grade level in math and reading. Generally, Ann was cooperative and a good worker in class, but there were occasions when she simply and completely refused to do an assigned task. At those times her classmates would rise to her defense and suggest, for instance, that Ann should still get a treat even if she didn't do her work.

To encourage more contact with others and active rather than passive communication of her needs and wishes, we began to implement a modified behavioral plan in the class. In the first stage of this plan, Ann was to raise her hand, tap the teacher, or signal in some identifiable way when she needs the teacher's attention. If over time Ann complied, our next step would be similar to one described by Halpern and colleagues (1971) in their behavioral approach to the symptom. This would be that Ann would select one word that she would say to the teacher in order, for example, to be released for recess. Regarding this point many authors note the importance of promptly stating the expectation that the child will speak and sharing that goal with the child, his or her classmates, and the staff.

Ann completed psychological testing during the fifth month after admission and the results bear mentioning. She showed an enormous variability in functioning and, depending upon the test administered, she scored from an average to a deficient I.Q. She performed better on concrete tasks than on those requiring abstract thinking, and her greatest weakness was in spatial orientation. Controlling and oppositional behavior as well as a fear of failure interfered with her ability to be fully cooperative in the testing. The possibility was raised that her mutism was used to cover areas of cognitive deficit.

I began seeing Ann in weekly individual psychotherapy shortly after her admission. At first she was reluctant to come into the office, though she had been in my office twice during the admission process. She spent our first session sitting outside my door. I remained in the office, wrote her a letter, and then played mailman and delivered it to her. This interchange had the effect of easing some of her anxiety, reducing her fears of intrusiveness, and setting an accepting, understanding climate for her. By the second session she entered the office but was still quite suspicious and grave in her expression. I drew a picture and sought her involvement only by asking her to pick out the colors I should use. She engaged with me in this process and gradually she lessened the physical distance that was between us and her stern mood softened.

In these first sessions, I introduced two of our goals of working together. One was that we would get to know each other better, and second that we would try to figure out how a girl could decide to stop talking.

By the third session her tentativeness and shyness were quite absent in her behavior. She walked freely into my office, commandeered my chair, and meticulously went through my desk. I wondered aloud if she was curious and wanted to know something about me. She also seemed worried about how and what I would uncover about her in our sessions.

Increasingly, Ann has taken on a more lively role in our sessions and this included more active attempts at pursuing communication. As an example, she showed an interest in my phone and began dialing random phone numbers. I capitalized on this by giving her the number for a recorded message of the time and weather. She frequently dialed this number and listened with intense interest as the temperature and time was repeated for her. I then suggested that I go to the office next door and she could call me. She nodded her agreement and dialed the number. She answered my simple questions with unintelligible whispers, the blowing of a whistle into the phone, and slamming the receiver on the desk. In response I commented that I could hear all the different sounds she knew how to make. In another session we made a tape recording as we played musical instruments together, and she took great pleasure in manipulating the recorder and making the sound come out.

Ann's play continued to express her wish to relate to and communicate with me. In our twelfth session, she sat outside my door and I was in the office. Four or five times she went through the following play sequence. She picked up a book from outside the office, laid it in front of my door, knocked on the door, and when I opened it she indicated that I should take the book into the office with me. As we went through the play, I interpreted that she was giving me gifts of other people's words and stories, and maybe she was wondering if someday she could give up her words and stories about herself. Again she silently closed the door, knocked on it, and as I opened it, instead of a book lying in front of the door, I found Ann. I picked her up as I had the books and commented that now she and all of her words and stories were inside the office with me. Her response to this was to send me next door to receive a phone call from her, and she uttered her first audible word to me, which was "What?"

In recent sessions, Ann began to show more hostility and distancing behavior toward me. She would sit across the room with a furious face and throw pipe cleaners at me. She would put yarn and other silly things in my hair and then laugh silently at me. It seemed that this behavior was an attempt to keep me at a distance, perhaps after feeling that she came too close. It likely also represented feelings in her own past of some type of emotional assault and humiliation at another's hands.

THE APPROACH TO INDIVIDUAL PSYCHOTHERAPY

At the risk of making an artificial distinction, it may be helpful for the purposes of this discussion to separate out the individual psychotherapy of these two cases from the backdrop of the intensive group and milieu work. This will serve to elucidate technique and to allow speculation on what factors within the psychotherapy produced change. The assumption should not be made that individual psychotherapy is sufficient to treat these children, but rather that the greatest benefit from the curative factors of psychotherapy can accrue when the treatment is interwoven in the fabric of a structured, supportive therapeutic day milieu.

A psychoanalytically informed approach to the treatment of both cases served as a foundation upon which obvious modifications of technique were required. Only a few basic assumptions could be made in beginning the therapy of these children. First, the mutism itself should not be the initial focus of intervention, for this would only serve to intensify controlling and oppositional defensive behavior and thus increase the silence. It would also be experienced, especially by the more disturbed child, as an invasive challenge to already fragile self-object boundaries. Second, the silence and all other mannerisms, expressions, and motor activity should be accepted and understood as communications worthy of exploration, clarification, or interpretation. Third, the therapist should be prepared to be quite flexible in his or her technique. This includes the types and frequency of interventions made, the place of therapy, and the therapist's use of him- or herself in the treatment hour.

In Paul's case a more formal approach to the treatment was possible because of his healthier ego structure and object relations. For example, sessions occurred almost exclusively within the therapist's office. Paul was able to tolerate that degree of closeness and when anxiety did surface, it was surmountable and did not require gross physical expressions, such as running out of the office. Additionally, more traditional interpretations could be made and used by Paul, especially as he began to feel more comfortable with verbal communication.

This was not the case with Ann. Buxbaum (1954) notes that in treating the child with tenuous object ties, the therapist must constantly be prepared to adjust to the child's fluctuating ego levels in order to reach him and that the therapist cannot proceed systematically as one could with a neurotically disturbed child. Ann represented just such a child and her therapy required the flexibility described. The day hospital building and much of the hospital campus were frequent sites for psychotherapy sessions as the confines of the office were too threatening for Ann and as her wish to explore her surroundings increased. I frequently functioned as a mother would in helping Ann explore the environment in a safe and protected manner. This helped to strengthen her reality testing and encourage contact with the world around her. Food was also a frequent part of the sessions and Ann's involvement of the therapist in obtaining and sharing a snack with her was encouraged as a step toward healthier object ties. Flexibility was constantly needed in the level of directive intervention by the therapist as well. At times, I would make suggestions for activities such as offering her a tape recorder if she appeared interested in making sounds. In other sessions, the time would be spent silently together without activity if this was what she needed. As Buxbaum indicates, the therapist of such children must be "more than interested in the patient." The therapist must be able to address whatever needs the child presents—to be held, fed, and so on.

In examining what factors may have fostered positive effects in the treatment of these children, there are several that bear mentioning. First is the extended duration of treatment with the same therapist. These children were afforded the opportunity for long-term intensive treatment with one therapist, permitting the development of trust, consistency, and stability in an object outside the isolated and constricted family. Second, the focus of therapy was on the child's defects in object relations, not on the mutism. With Ann in particular, the relationship to the therapist was a major part of the therapy. Third, the child was not removed from the home. This permitted the child an optimal distance to work on the overly dependent relationship with the mother through daily contact with the therapist and other clinical staff members.

In conclusion, the day hospital work with these two children has been a combination of intensive psychotherapy, behavioral techniques, milieu therapy, and group treatment. I feel that it is this combination that can make for a lasting removal of the symptoms based on a working through of the underlying conflicts. Though I think the involvement of the family in treatment can, in some cases, speed the therapeutic process, I do not feel it is essential nor should it be demanded as a condition for treating the child. In Paul's case, I would offer that the family's refusal to work intensely with us gave him the needed distance from this engulfing, closed-off family, to separate and become an individual both in and outside of the family.

In our work with both these children we have tried to move speech from the realm of anxiety-producing behavior to that of anxiety-reducing behavior. The two case examples of our therapeutic approaches toward this end illuminate the road for those clinicians who take on the work of these challenging, silent children.

REFERENCES

Adams, H., and Glasner, P. (1954). Emotional involvements in some forms of mutism. *Journal of Speech and Hearing Disorders* 19:59–69.

American Psychiatric Association. (1980). *Diagnostic and Statistical Manual of Mental Disorders, Third Edition (DSM-III)*. Washington, DC: American Psychiatric Association.

Amman, H. (1958). Schweigende Kinder. *Heilpadagogik Werkbl.* 27:209–216.

Arlow, J. A. (1961). Silence and the theory of technique. *Journal of the American Psychoanalytic Association* 9:44–55.

Blos, P. (1972). Silence: a clinical exploration. *Psychoanalytic Quarterly* 41:348–363.

Bradley, S., and Sloman, L. (1975). Elective mutism in immigrant families. *Journal of the American Academy of Child Psychiatry* 14:510–514.

Browne, E., Wilson, V., and Laybourne, P. (1963). Diagnosis in treatment of elective mutism in children. *Journal of the American Academy of Child Psychiatry* 2:605–617.

Chapin, A. B., and Corcoran, N. (1947). A program for the speech inhibited child. *Journal of Speech and Hearing Disorders* 12:373–376.

Chethik, M. (1973). Amy: the intensive treatment of an elective mute. *Journal of the American Academy of Child Psychiatry* 12:482–498.

Edgcumbe, R. (1981). Toward a developmental line for the acquisition of language. *Psychoanalytic Study of the Child* 36:71–103. New Haven, CT: Yale University Press.

Elson, A., Pearson, C., Jones, C. D., and Schumacher, E. (1965). Follow-up study of childhood elective mutism. *Archives of General Psychiatry* 13:182–187.

Glover, E. (1955). *The Technique of Psychoanalysis.* New York: International Universities Press.

Goll, K. (1979). Role structure and subculture in families of elective mutists. *Family Process* 18:55–68.

Halpern, W., Hammond, J., and Cohen, R. (1971). A therapeutic approach to speech phobia: elective mutism re-examined. *Journal of the American Academy of Child Psychiatry* 10:94–107.

Hayden, T. L. (1980). Classification of elective mutism. *Journal of the American Academy of Child Psychiatry* 19:118–133.

Kahn, M. (1963). Silence as communication. *Bulletin of the Menninger Clinic* 27:300–313.

Kehrer, H. E., and Tinkl-Damhorst, N. (1974). Verhaltensterapie bie elektivem mutismus. *Acta Paedopsychiatrica* 41:34–44.

Kolvin, I., and Fundudis, T. (1981). Elective mute children: psychological development and background factors. *Journal of Child Psychology and Psychiatry* 22:219–232.

Kummer, R. (1953). Betrachtungen zum problem des freiwilligen schweigens. *Psychiatrie, Neurologie, and Medizinische Psychologie* 5:79–83.

Kupietz, S., and Schwartz, I. (1982). Elective mutism. Evaluation and behavioral treatment of three cases. *State Journal of Medicine* 82:1073–1076.

Miller, R. (1979). Language acquisition. *Basic Handbook of Child Psychiatry* 1:127–143.

Mitscherlich, M. (1961). Zwei falle von psychogenem mutismus. *Zeitschrift fur Psychosomatische Medizin* 7:172–175.

Mora, G., Devautt, S., and Schopler, E. (1962). Dynamics and psychotherapy of identical twins with elective mutism. *Journal of Child Psychology and Psychiatry* 7:41–52.

Parker, E. B., Olsen, T. F., and Throckmorton, M. C. (1960). Social casework with elementary school children who do not talk in school. *Social Work* 5:64–70.

Pine, F. (1984). The interpretive moment: variations on classical themes. *Bulletin of the Menninger Clinic* 48:54–71.

Pustrom, E., and Speers, R. W. (1964). Elective mutism in children. *Journal of the American Academy of Child Psychiatry* 3:287–297.

Reed, G. F. (1963). Elective mutism in children: a reappraisal. *Journal of Child Psychology and Psychiatry* 4:99–107.

Ruzicka, B., and Sackin, H. (1974). Elective mutism. The impact of the patient's silent detachment upon the therapist. *Journal of the American Academy of Child Psychiatry* 13:551–561.

Salfield, D. J. (1950). Observations on elective mutism in children. *Journal of Mental Science* 96:1024–1032.

Spieler, J. (1944). *Schweigende und Sprachschewe Kinder*. Olten: Walter.

Thomas, A., Chess, S., and Birch, H. G. (1968). *Temperament and Behavior Disorders in Children*. New York: New York University Press.

von Misch, A. (1952). Elektiver mutismus im Kindersalter. *Zeitschrift fur Kinderpsychiatrie* 19:49–87.

Waterink, J., and Vedder, R. (1936). Einige falle von thymogenem mutismus bei sehr jungen kindern und seine behandlung. *Zeitschrift fur Kinderforschung* 45:368–369.

Weissman, M. (1982). Unpublished paper on elective mutism.

Wergeland, H. (1979). Elective mutism. *Acta Psychiatrica Scandinavica* 59:218–228.

Wright, H. (1968). A clinical study of children who refuse to talk. *Journal of the American Academy of Child Psychiatry* 7:603–617.

Yates, A. J. (1970). *Behavior Therapy*. New York: Wiley.

Zeligs, M. (1961). The psychology of silence. Its role in transference, counter-transference and psychoanalytic process. *Journal of the American Psychoanalytic Association* 9:7–43.

17

CASE STUDY: FLUOXETINE IN THE MULTIMODAL TREATMENT OF A PRESCHOOL CHILD WITH SELECTIVE MUTISM

Harry H. Wright, Michael L. Cuccaro,
Tami V. Leonhardt, Dorothy F. Kendall,
and Julie H. Anderson

SELECTIVE MUTISM IS a rare disorder of childhood character-ized by consistent failure to speak in specific social situations despite speaking in other situations. The disturbance interferes with educa-tional achievement and social communication (American Psychiat-ric Association 1994). Prevalence rates for selective mutism of 0.3 to 0.8 per 1,000 have been reported (Brown and Lloyd 1975, Fundudis et al. 1979). Onset of the disorder is usually in the preschool years, but the average age of referral and diagnosis is between 6 and 8 years (Krohn et al. 1992, Wright et al. 1985). A higher incidence in fe-males has been reported (Black and Uhde 1992).

Factors associated with selective mutism include excessive shy-ness, oppositional/manipulative behavior, mental retardation, speech disorder, hospitalization/trauma before age 3 years, maternal over-protection, parental conflict, and family immigration/isolation (Bra-dley and Sloman 1975, Browne et al. 1963, Klin and Volkmar 1993, Krohn et al. 1992, Parker et al. 1960, Wilkins 1985, Wright 1968). Appropriate classification of this disorder has been debated for at least the last decade (Black and Uhde 1992, Wilkins 1985). Some authors argue that selective mutism is a variant of social phobia (Black and Uhde 1992), while others focus on the relationship of selective mutism to panic disorder and separation anxiety disorder (Golwyn and Weinstock 1990, Lesser-Katz 1988, Wilkins 1985) or oppositional/controlling behaviors (Krohn et al. 1992).

Most of the literature on selective mutism consists of single-case reports or small case series. Among these reports, a wide range of treatment strategies has been described (Wright et al. 1994) including individual, group, and family approaches. Treatment outcomes have been inconclusive at best (Krohn et al. 1992, Wright et al. 1985). In fact, Wergeland (1979) observed a better outcome in an untreated group of children with selective mutism versus a treated group. Krohn and colleagues (1992) concluded that behavioral approaches to treatment were generally more effective than purely dynamic interventions. Most recently there have been reports of pharmacological treatment of selective mutism in two school-age children (Black and Uhde 1992, Golwyn and Weinstock 1990). In both cases there was dramatic improvement in the selective mutism.

Treating selective mutism presents great challenges. The optimal intervention strategy may be a comprehensive, multifaceted therapeutic approach (Hechtman 1993). However, few reports have focused on a multimodal treatment approach (Wright et al. 1994). This chapter describes the treatment of a preschool girl with selective mutism and her family via a multimodal approach that includes family therapy, behavioral therapy, play therapy, and pharmacotherapy.

CASE STUDY

HISTORY

"Leah F." was a 4-year, 10-month-old white girl who presented to the outpatient clinic for evaluation for failure to speak in social situations outside her home for more than seven months. Leah attended nursery school, where she had been talking freely with nursery staff and peers until her mother increased her work schedule from two to three days a week. Leah's mother responded to her failure to speak in school by cutting back her work schedule. At home, Leah continued to be quite talkative and had no apparent difficulties with speech and language. Outside of the home, Leah would sometimes communicate through nonverbal means, using facial expressions and gestures and nodding or shaking her head; frequently, however, she refused to talk at all.

Leah attended another preschool program three months after she stopped talking. She never spoke at her new preschool program even when her parents arrived, but she did speak to her parents when they left the building. She often greeted them by saying, "I didn't speak at all today." When asked why, she frequently answered either, "Because I want to go to work with Mommy" or "I was too shy."

Leah was born after seven years of her parents' marriage. The pregnancy, labor, and delivery were without difficulties. Leah said her first words at approximately 12 months, but she did not begin walking until 14 or 15 months. Toilet training was described as very difficult because of episodic bouts of constipation. Leah's mother admits that she was overprotective.

There is no family history of selective mutism, communication difficulties, or mental retardation. Leah's mother reports that she was slow to "warm up" as an infant and young child and was afraid of teachers and authority figures as a school-age child. She reports she is shy and somewhat socially phobic as an adult.

TREATMENT COURSE

Nine months after she stopped talking, Leah and her family started treatment in an outpatient preschool diagnostic and intervention day program (Miller et al. 1982, Wright et al. 1985). During the initial assessment Leah's mother completed the Child Behavior Checklist (CBCL) and Parenting Stress Index (PSI), and served as the informant for the Vineland Adaptive Behavioral Scales (VABS).

On entering the program, Leah appeared to be uninterested in and avoidant of social interaction. She had difficulty separating from her parents and often hid her face in her hands when approached by program staff. During the first week she gritted her teeth at staff, clenched her fists, and held her body rigid. When required, she would sit with the group during activities and snack time but refused to participate. When her oppositional behavior resulted in time-out, she often refused to rejoin the group afterward.

Leah gradually became less oppositional, appeared less anxious, and was generally more socially responsive. She began to shadow a staff member and used her as a secure base from which to venture into the larger environment of the playroom and outside play space. Leah became frustrated and withdrew if a staff member did not follow her lead. She gradually interacted cautiously with peers and relied less on adults. Separating from her parents each morning was no longer problematic by week 7. Also she initiated contact with staff and peers through gestures (i.e., pointing to desired play items) by week 9.

The parents participated in a weekly parent group and were also seen in individual and couple sessions. Leah participated in individual play sessions twice a week. Specific behavioral approaches were discussed with the parents and were initiated in the day program and at home. Home and school visits were made.

Leah was still not talking at the end of the twelve-week program but appeared considerably less anxious and oppositional. She remained controlling in situations where she was anxious (i.e., when staff asked her to complete a task). At this point Leah and her family were seen on a weekly basis in outpatient treatment. Leah's behavioral intervention was continued and extended to Leah's public school kindergarten.

Despite positive changes in several areas, Leah was still not talking after six months of treatment. It was decided in consultation with parents to add a trial of medication.

After a physical examination by her pediatrician, electrocardiogram, laboratory studies, and written consent by parents, Leah began fluoxetine therapy. The initial dosage of 4 mg/day was increased to 8 mg/day by twelve days. Leah began to talk more freely in familiar settings after five days of fluoxetine treatment and by day 20 of treatment, she was talking freely in all settings. However, her oppositional behavior increased as she talked more.

Leah had a successful summer during which she continued to talk freely in all settings. She is repeating kindergarten because she was very immature socially, but the current school year has gone very well, with Leah making considerable academic and behavioral progress. At the first reporting period, the teacher's only comment was that "Leah could do better if she did not talk so much." Leah's mother increased her work schedule to three days a week without difficulty.

Leah reports that she was "shy" and "afraid to talk," but not now. One year after beginning fluoxetine therapy, she continues to take the drug. She has not experienced any adverse medication effects. Leah's medication is monitored and the family continues in family therapy on a monthly basis.

FORMAL ASSESSMENT RESULTS

The initial (time 1) assessments (CBCL, PSI, and VABS) were repeated eighteen months later (time 2) (Tables 17-1 to 17-3). On the CBCL there was a clear reduction in internalizing symptoms at time 2 assessment. Problem behaviors shifted from clinically significant to borderline significant. Several changes across time were noted including a reduction in withdrawal and somatic complaints. At the same time, there was an increase in behavior problems associated with social difficulties.

Overall levels of problem behavior on the PSI remained the same. However, there was a reduction in Leah's mood-related and adaptability difficulties and an increase in motor activity and distractibility. Mrs. F.'s perception of restriction of role secondary to her child's difficulties were also reduced. However, the depression subdomain was in the borderline clinically significant range at both times.

Table 17–1.
Child Behavior Checklist Ratings: T Scores

	Time 1	Time 2
Total problem score	66[a]	64
Internalizing	68[a]	60
Externalizing	54	58
Withdrawn	68[a]	61
Somatic complaints	67[a]	54
Anxious/depressed	61	63
Social problems	62	70[a]
Thought problems	58	58
Attention problems	66	66
Delinquent behavior	51	51
Aggressive behavior	55	59

[a]Clinically significant scores.

Table 17–2.
Parenting Stress Index Scores

	Time 1	Time 2
Summary scores		
Total	274[a]	270[a]
Child domain	115	116
Parent domain	159[a]	154[a]
Child domain		
Adaptability	35[a]	30
Acceptability	13	14
Demandingness	20[a]	20
Mood	16	11
Distractibility/hyperactivity	24	34[a]
Reinforces parent	7	7
Parent domain		
Depression	26	24
Attachment	12	12
Restriction of role	26[a]	12
Sense of competence	35	33
Social isolation	22[a]	20[a]

Table 17–2. Continued.
Parenting Stress Index Scores

	Time 1	Time 2
Relationship spouse	29[a]	29[a]
Parent health	9	11

[a]Clinically significant scores.

Table 17–3.
Adaptive Behavior Ratings

	Standard Scores/Age Equivalents for Adaptive Behavior Composite and Domain Scores			
	Time 1		Time 2	
	Mean ± SD	Year-Month	Mean ± SD	Year-Month
Adaptive behavior composite	71 ± 6		64 ± 5	
Communication	92 ± 8	4-7	74 ± 7	4-10
Daily living skills	72 ± 9	3-5	59 ± 8	4-1
Socialization	81 ± 10	3-6	74 ± 8	4-2
Motor skills[a]	63 ± 13	3-4	78 ± 13	4-8

	Age-Equivalent Scores for Subdomains: Year-Month	
	Time 1	Time 2
Receptive	3-11	3-11
Expressive	5-06	5-09
Written	4-01	4-08
Personal	3-03	3-03
Domestic	3-09	3-06
Community	3-04	4-02
Interpersonal relationships	4-10	5-03
Play and leisure time	2-04	3-10
Coping skills	3-07	3-10
Gross motor skills	4-07	4-07
Fine motor skills	2-09	4-09

[a]Estimated at time 2.

Leah's adaptive behaviors on the VABS did not keep pace with age-expected changes. Nonetheless, there were slight gains when age equivalents were inspected. Leah's cognitive abilities were in the average range.

DISCUSSION

Various treatment approaches have been suggested for selective mutism. Most have not proven to be very effective. Whereas only a few reports have described multimodal interventions with selective mutism in children (Krohn et al. 1992, Wright et al. 1985, 1994), the combination of treatment approaches appears to have more promise for effective intervention in a difficult-to-treat disorder. The approach used in this case adds a psychopharmacological intervention to a previously described multimodal approach (Wright et al. 1985). To our knowledge only two other case reports have described a psychopharmacological intervention as part of the treatment for selective mutism (Black and Uhde 1992, Golwyn and Weinstock 1990). Some of the characteristics of this case and the two others that used a psychopharmacological component are summarized in Table 17–4.

Table 17–4.
Psychoactive Medication in Selective Mutism

Study	Age at Referral	Age at Onset	History of Shyness	Family History of Anxiety Disorder	Length of Treatment before Medication	Medication
Golwyn and Weinstock (1990)	7 yr	5 yr	Yes	Yes	4 mo	Phenelzine 52.5 mg/d
Black and Uhde (1992)	12 yr	5 yr	Yes	Yes	> 12 mo	Fluoxetine 20 mg/d
This report	5 yr	4 yr	Yes	Yes	12 mo	Fluoxetine 8 mg/d

Leah had a typical circumstance and age of onset for selective mutism (Krohn et al. 1992, Wright et al. 1985). The associated features of prominent anxiety and oppositionalism demonstrated in this case have been described as well (Black and Uhde 1992, Krohn et al. 1992). Leah's anxiety was not initially recognized in the presence of moderate to severe oppositional behavior. In the absence of other coping strategies, Leah relied on oppositional behavior to control her interaction with others and contain her anxiety. There was a clear family history of anxiety disorder.

We have argued that early intervention with children with selective mutism results in more effective treatment and better outcomes. In addition, having a wide range of interventions available to select the most appropriate treatment combinations for each individual may also improve the prognosis (Wright et al. 1985). For example, the addition of the psychopharmacological intervention to family, play, and behavioral therapy in this case led to Leah's speaking in settings where she had been mute for more than one-and-a-half years. The use of the medication may have facilitated a reduction in inhibition (anxiety), resulting in Leah's ability to perform (talk) with minimal stress. As in social phobia, the effectiveness of fluoxetine in this case is thought to be due to the antianxiety rather than the antidepressant effects. A child with selective mutism may be overcontrolled/inhibited. Medication may allow the child to be available to learn and execute skills acquired in other modalities (i.e., play or behavior therapy).

The psychosocial components of the multimodal treatment focused on specific problem areas. We have generally begun with behaviorally based interventions with parents and teachers and play therapy with the child. Adult care providers are taught to avoid inadvertent reinforcement of the child's mutism and to expect and reinforce speech efforts. Play therapy is directed toward increasing a sense of the child's competence and independence while decreasing anxiety. Behavioral therapy is focused on increasing the consistency of responses to communicating and providing limits and structure across settings. Family and couple therapy may affect family structure and function, including child-rearing practices and family roles. In cases where anxiety appears salient and psychosocial therapies do not produce appreciable gains, the use of medication should be considered.

The conceptualization of selective mutism as a variant of social anxiety leads one to consider medications that have been effectively used in anxiety disorders (Marshall et al. 1994). As anxiety is reduced, one may see an initial increase in oppositional behaviors, which the family and behavioral therapy can address.

Several issues emerged in the use of the formal assessment instruments to evaluate ongoing symptomatology and monitor treatment.

First, parent ratings generally do not provide a detailed picture of change in anxiety and mood symptoms. However, clinically significant changes occurred over time in this case. A focused assessment of internalizing symptoms may yield a better picture of the child's difficulties and changes.

A second consideration involves the influence of parental anxiety and depressive symptoms on child ratings. For example, Mrs. F.'s ratings of Leah's behavior may reflect changes in her own anxiety and depressive symptoms. However, Mrs. F. did not report changes (i.e., depression, marital relations, or sense of isolation).

A third issue involves the assessment of behavior problems via parent report in children with selective mutism. Typically, children with selective mutism exhibit markedly different language and communication behaviors in the home environment versus public or nonhome environments. The extent to which other behaviors differ across settings is not known. For example, oppositional behaviors are frequently observed in children with selective mutism (Wright and Cuccaro 1994). As a correlate of selective mutism, this behavior may also differ across settings. Clearly, this point highlights the importance of multimethod assessment across settings and situations for selectively mute children.

This case illustrates the importance of early identification, comprehensive assessment, and multimodal intervention in the treatment of young children with selective mutism. The components of this intervention reflect a conceptualization of selective mutism that emphasizes anxiety as a core feature. The impact of selective mutism on others is highlighted. Further research with a larger number of preschool children with selective mutism may continue to clarify the issues raised in this report.

REFERENCES

American Psychiatric Association. (1994). *Diagnostic and Statistical Manual of Mental Disorders, Fourth Edition (DSM-IV)*. Washington, DC: American Psychiatric Association.

Black, M., and Uhde, T. W. (1992). Elective mutism as a variant of social phobia. *Journal of the American Academy of Child and Adolescent Psychiatry* 31:711-718.

Bradley, S., and Sloman, L. (1975). Elective mutism in immigrant families. *Journal of the American Academy of Child Psychiatry* 14:510-514.

Brown, J. B., and Lloyd, H. (1975). A controlled study of children not speaking at school. *Journal of the Associated Workers for Maladjusted Children* 3:49-63.

Browne, E., Wilson, V., and Laybourne, P. C. (1963). Diagnosis and treatment of elective mutism in children. *Journal of the American Academy of Child Psychiatry* 2:605-617.

Fundudis, T., Kolvin, I., and Garside, R. (1979). *Speech Retarded and Deaf Children: Their Psychological Development*. London: Academic Press.

Golwyn, D. H., and Weinstock, R. C. (1990). Phenelzine treatment of elective mutism. *Journal of Clinical Psychiatry* 51:384-385.

Hechtman, L. (1993). Aims and methodological problems in multimodal treatment studies. *Canopy of Journal Psychiatry* 38:458-464.

Klin, A., and Volkmar, F. R. (1993). Elective mutism and mental retardation. *Journal of the American Academy of Child and Adolescent Psychiatry* 32:860-864.

Krohn, D. D., Weckstein, S. M., and Wright, H. L. (1992). A study of the effectiveness of a specific treatment for elective mutism. *Journal of the American Academy of Child and Adolescent Psychiatry* 31:711–718.

Lesser-Katz, M. (1988). The treatment of elective mutism as stranger reaction. *Psychotherapy* 25:305–313.

Marshall, R. D., Schnier, F. R., Fallon, B. A., et al. (1994). Medication therapy for social phobia. *Journal of Clinical Psychiatry* 55 (suppl.):33–37.

Miller, M. D., Wright, H. H., and Hamilton, C. (1982). A teaching hospital-based diagnostic nursery program. *North Carolina Journal of Mental Health* 9:37–41.

Parker, E. B., Elsen, T. F., and Throckmorton, M. C. (1960). Social casework with elementary school children who do not talk in school. *Social Casework* 5:64–70.

Wergeland, H. (1979). Elective mutism. *Acta Psychiatrica Scandinavica* 59:218–228.

Wilkins, R. (1985). A comparison of elective mutism and emotional disorder in children. *British Journal of Psychiatry* 146:198–203.

Wright, H. H., and Cuccaro, M. I. (1994). Selective mutism continued. *Journal of the American Academy of Child and Adolescent Psychiatry* 33:593–594.

Wright, H. H., Holmes, G. R., Cuccaro, M. L., and Leonhardt, T. V. (1994). A guided bibliography of the selective mutism (elective mutism) literature. *Psychological Reports* 74:995–1007.

Wright, H. H., Miller, M. D., Cook, M. A., and Littmann, J. R. (1985). Early identification and intervention with children who refuse to speak. *Journal of the American Academy of Child Psychiatry* 24:739–746.

Wright, H. L. (1968). A clinical study of children who refuse to talk in school. *Journal of the American Academy of Child Psychiatry* 7:603–617.

CREDITS

INDEX

ABOUT THE EDITORS

Sheila A. Spasaro, Ph.D., is a clinical psychologist with the Rockland County, New York Chapter of NYSARC, and maintains a consulting psychology practice in Dutchess County, NY. She is a former adjunct faculty member at Fairleigh Dickinson University in Teaneck, New Jersey, and Drew University in Madison, NJ. Dr. Spasaro is co-author of "Infant Night Waking" in C. E. Schaefer's *Clinical Handbook of Sleep Disorders in Children* (1995), and has presented and published numerous professional articles.

Charles E. Schaefer, Ph.D., is Professor of Psychology and Director, Psychological Services Center, Fairleigh Dickinson University, Hackensack, New Jersey. Dr. Schaefer is the founder and Chairman of the Board of the Association for Play Therapy. He is a Fellow of both the American Psychological Association and the American Orthopsychiatric Association. Among Dr. Schaefer's publications are the outstanding books *Handbook of Play Therapy* and *The Therapeutic Use of Child's Play*, which have become classics in the field. Dr. Schaefer maintains a private practice with children and families in Hackensack.